HEALTH MATTERS

A Pocket Guide to Working with Diverse Cultures and Underserved Populations

D0710828

Praise for *Health Matters*

"The cultural makeup of the U.S. is changing. With that change comes the need for tools to help us understand what appears to be different from the norm, especially in areas of the country that were culturally homogeneous and now experience fundamental shifts. *Health Matters* provides a much-needed tool to assist with that understanding."

— Janice Edmunds-Wells, Consultant, Office of Multicultural Health, Iowa Dept. of Public Health

"*Health Matters* is a very important book for understanding cultural factors. Dr. Yehieli and Dr. Grey offer distinctive solutions and ways to approach working with minority groups in the United States. The authors take great care to explain the uniqueness of each individual human being, showing how social and cultural forces shape us individually and ultimately affect the way we approach health. It is a good tool for health providers to have on hand to better understand the role of culture in shaping health. Health Matters is also excellent reading material for students interested in working with diverse peoples."

— Osman Galal, M.D., Ph.D., Professor and Director, International Health Program, UCLA School of Public Health

"As the United States continues its dramatic demographic shifts, health care providers struggle to understand and care effectively for newcomers and diverse patient populations. A strong addition for your cross-cultural health care library, this outstanding guide provides practical and succinct information to practitioners working with refugees, immigrants and other underserved populations. A must-read for those truly committed to reducing health disparities in a multicultural nation."

— Patricia F. Walker, M.D., DTM&H, Medical Director, HealthPartners Center for International Health

HEALTH MATTERS

A Pocket Guide to Working with Diverse Cultures and Underserved Populations

Michele Yehieli, Dr. P.H., and Mark A. Grey, Ph.D.

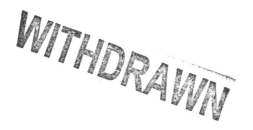

INTERCULTURAL PRESS
A Nicholas Brealey Publishing Company

YARMOUTH, ME • BOSTON • LONDON

First published by Intercultural Press, a Nicholas Brealey Publishing Company, in 2005.

Intercultural Press, a division of Nicholas Brealey Publishing
100 City Hall Plaza, Ste. 501
Boston, MA 02108
Information: 617-523-3801
Fax: 617-523-3708
www.interculturalpress.com

Nicholas Brealey Publishing
3-5 Spafield Street, Clerkenwell
London, EC1R 4QB, UK
Tel: +44-(0)-207-239-0360
Fax: +44-(0)-207-239-0370
www.nbrealey-books.com

Cover and text design by Lisa Garbutt, Rara Avis Graphic Design

Printed in the United States of America

09 08 07 06 05   1 2 3 4 5

ISBN: 1-931930-20-1

It is much more important to know what kind of person has a disease, than what kind of disease a person has.

—*Sir William Osler*

CONTENTS

ACKNOWLEDGMENTS.. ix
INTRODUCTION xi

**Part 1: The Immigrant, Refugee, and Minority Health Care
Experience in the United States...................... 1**
America's Changing Ethnic Landscape.................... 1
Challenges for Health Care Providers and Minorities,
Immigrants, and Refugees 2

Part 2: Culturally Appropriate Health Care 8
Defining Culture.. 8
Categorizing Culture Groups............................ 9
Cultural Communication Styles 11

**Part 3: Becoming More Culturally Appropriate:
General Strategies................................... 13**
Guidelines for Providers 13
Making Health Organizations More Accommodating 16
Public Health Planning for Newcomer Populations 19
Working Effectively with Interpreters................. 22
Working with Low-Literacy Patients 25
Understanding Traditional Health Practices........... 26

Part 4: The Cultural Communities 31
African Americans...................................... 33
The Amish 40
Arab Muslims 46
Bosnian Refugees 54
East African Refugees................................. 60

East Asian Immigrants 69

Hispanics 77

Indians. 87

Iranians 94

Jews 100

Native Americans 109

Pacific Islanders 119

Russians and Eastern Europeans 125

Southeast Asian Refugees 131

Part 5: Resources 137

National Resources on Minority, Immigrant,
    and Refugee Health. 137

National Resources on Minority Aging Issues. 140

Recommended Readings on Minority,
    Immigrant, and Refugee Health 142

References and Other Resources. 143

The Iowa Project EXPORT Center of Excellence
    on Health Disparities. 144

The Iowa Center for Immigrant Leadership
    and Integration 145

ABOUT THE AUTHORS. 146

ACKNOWLEDGMENTS

We would like to acknowledge and thank many University of Northern Iowa (UNI) administrators and faculty for their support of the Iowa Project EXPORT Center of Excellence on Health Disparities, the Iowa Center for Immigration Leadership and Integration, the Global Health Corps, and the New Iowans Program. They include UNI President Dr. Robert Koob; Dr. Patricia Geadelmann, Special Assistant to the President for Board and Governmental Relations; Keith Saunders, Associate Director of Governmental Relations; Dr. Susan Koch, Associate Vice President of Academic Affairs; Dr. Aaron Podolefsky, Provost; Dr. Julia Wallace, Dean of the College of Social and Behavioral Sciences; Dr. Christopher Edginton, Director of the School of Health, Physical Education, and Leisure Services; Dr. Sue Joslyn, Professor of Health Education; Dr. Gene Lutz, Director of the UNI Center for Social and Behavioral Research; and Dr. Anne Woodrick, Associate Professor of Anthropology. We also express our gratitude to our staff members, including Jan Cornelius, Annie Vander Werff, Linda K. Miller, Nora Rodriguez, Abbie Peterson, and Mary Bellone Grey.

The authors would especially like to thank the following professionals from the cultural communities discussed in this guidebook for their invaluable assistance as reviewers: the Black Hawk County Minority Health Coalition, the Cedar Valley Hospice (Stacey Taylor and Tina Hubbard), Dr. Roberto Clemente, Eileen Corcoran, Dr.

Robin Gurien, Dr. Yulia Komarova, Nora Rodriguez, Yana Cornish, Patricia Teran Yengle, Dr. Sang-Min Kim, Clementine and Israel Msengi, Dr. Rahdi Al-Mabuk, John Sagala, Dr. Christina Thomas, Hagai Yehieli, Janice Edmunds-Well, Peladija Woodson, Dr. Catherine Zeman, and Dr. Douglas Zhu.

A shorter version of this book was produced as part of the outreach and training efforts of the Iowa Project EXPORT Center of Excellence on Health Disparities and the Iowa Center for Immigrant Leadership and Integration, including the New Iowans Program. These programs represent the University of Northern Iowa's commitment to welcoming immigrant and refugee newcomers to the United States, and helping to address the needs of longtime minority populations as well.

Finally, we wish to acknowledge the love and support we receive from our families: Hagai and Daniel Yehieli, and Mary, Megan, and Julia Cameron Grey. Without them, our work at the University of Northern Iowa to address health disparities and other critical issues facing minorities, immigrants, and refugees would not be possible.

INTRODUCTION

This pocket guide is a practical resource for health care, social work, public health, and related providers who work with the growing number of immigrants, refugees, and minorities in the United States. These populations typically experience unique cultural, social, and economic barriers that can significantly affect their health status. Working with diverse populations can be very rewarding, but it can also pose a number of challenges for hospitals, clinics, county health departments, Medicare organizations, nonprofit organizations, social service agencies, and other entities that serve these groups.

This book was developed in response to a growing demand among physicians, nurses, educators, community health workers, and other caring professionals for information and practical advice on how to work with newcomer and minority populations. The information provided in this guide comes from a number of different sources as cited in the reference section, as well as from the extensive backgrounds of the authors, who have decades of academic and field experience working directly with immigrants, refugees, and minorities around the world. Other sources of information for this book include the body of professional health literature and the knowledge of many providers who have shared their experiences with us. Most important, clients and professionals from each of the minority populations have provided extensive input.

In the late 1990s, we started two major programs at the University of Northern Iowa to address the unique health and other needs of Iowa's rapidly growing minority, immigrant, and refugee populations: the Global Health Corps and the New Iowans Program. Iowa remains a predominately white state, but a growing number of communities are experiencing major influxes of immigrants and refugees. We recognized the unique challenges these newcomers brought to Iowa communities, health care providers, and workplaces. We started the Global Health Corps and New Iowans Program to address the unique needs of minorities and newcomers, but we soon recognized an even greater demand among health care providers, social workers, employers, community leaders, and others for basic, readily available information about these groups and how to effectively work with them. We also frequently provided training to health care providers in a variety of institutional settings on how to effectively work with minority and immigrant populations.

As the breadth and depth of the Global Health Corps and the New Iowans Program changed and grew, we established two larger, more inclusive centers: The Iowa Project EXPORT Center of Excellence on Health Disparities and the Iowa Center for Immigrant Leadership and Integration. The EXPORT (Excellence in Partnerships for Outreach, Research, and Training) Center on Health Disparities is part of a national system of such organizations funded by the National Center on Minority Health and Health Disparities at the National Institutes of Health. As a result of our increasing role in addressing multicultural needs, our organizations began to write and publish a series of handbooks for Iowa providers and others. For example, we published a series of books under the major title *Welcoming New Iowans*, including books for communities and citizens, churches, and the workplace. Additional titles were produced to address health care issues, including our *A Health Provider's Pocket Guide to Working with Immigrant, Refugee, and Minority Patients in Iowa; Caring for Diverse Seniors: A Health Provider's Pocket Guide to Working with Elderly Minority, Immigrant, and Refugee Patients; Reaching Out to Elderly Minorities, Immigrants, and Refugees: A Senior Medicare Patrol Pocket Guide; and Orthodox Jewish Patients in Hospital Settings: A Health Provider's Pocket Guide.*

This current book, *Health Matters*, is therefore a new, expanded guide that includes material that was previously published in the above series of books. *Health Matters* was written in response to a growing demand for information found in our previous guidebooks for Iowa, but put in a single volume that addresses the health care and other needs of minorities, immigrants, and refugees throughout the United States. Our experience writing, producing, and distributing similar guides made it abundantly clear to us that there is a tremendous demand for quick, easily accessible information on how to work with diverse cultures and underserved populations. We also recognized that a growing number of our publications were going to communities, governments, and institutions outside Iowa. This reflects, of course, the growing demand for information and training about working with minorities, immigrants, and refugees throughout a changing United States. Indeed, as we describe in Part 1, the U.S. is experiencing tremendous demographic changes with growth among minority and immigrant populations that far outstrips that of the nation's white population. The political discourse about immigration and major population shifts ebbs and flows, but regardless of the politics, the health care and social service needs of minorities and newcomers present very real challenges to health care and other personnel. We wrote *Health Matters* exactly for these people who have to make the new demographic and cultural reality work at the ground level.

FOCUS OF THIS BOOK

This guide responds to several questions:

1. What are the cultural backgrounds of some of the most significant minority and newcomer populations in the United States?

2. How do the cultural, religious, and socioeconomic backgrounds of these groups impact their perspectives on health and the

health care system? How do patients and clients from different cultures define *health*?

3. What should health care providers know about these minorities and newcomers that will help them provide the best possible care?

We address these questions in five sections. Part 1 provides background information on the changing ethnic landscape in the United States, as well as introductory material on the critical challenges these demographic shifts present to care providers and minority patients. In Part 2, we discuss the key concepts associated with culturally appropriate health care, including an introduction to human culture and cultural communication styles. Part 3 provides detailed instruction on how individuals and institutions can develop culturally appropriate service strategies. This section also includes some hands-on advice on working with interpreters and low-literacy patients.

In Part 4, we provide information on a number of minority, immigrant, refugee, and other diverse and underserved populations. In this section, we address some of the specific key differences among these groups, and how these cultural and ethnic experiences shape their ideas about health, the health care system in the United States, and how to access it. We want to emphasize, however, that although this guide provides valuable information about the best ways to approach health issues for patients and clients from individual ethnic groups, it is not meant to stereotype any person. Health providers must recognize the tremendous diversity among individual practices, beliefs, and personalities of all patients, regardless of their countries of origin or ethnicities.

Finally, in Part 5, we provide lists of key institutions and resources as well as some critical reading materials on minority, immigrant, and refugee health.

We purposefully kept this book short in order to create a relatively small and easily accessible guide to working with these unique populations. This approach also grew out of our experience with our previous publications and in our training of health care and other professionals. We recognize our readers are busy people who don't have time to sit down and read textbooks every time they work with new populations. In addition to getting to the point and providing information that is easy to find, we know from our experience that the guide must be portable, and thus the small format.

By their very nature, books of this kind can only provide guidance and advice. We provide snapshots of the different cultures that give a basis for understanding how patients and clients from these ethnic and national groups may conceptualize health and how they view institutions such as clinics and hospitals. Ultimately, of course, all patients and clients are unique people, and despite their propensity to speak certain languages or have different, culturally based views on life, they are still individuals and they must be treated as such. Indeed, we emphasize in our publications and training that all health and service providers recognize the tremendous variation *within* cultures and populations as well as *among* different cultures and populations.

The quote we provide as the epigraph to this book from Sir William Osler is worth repeating here:

It is much more important to know what kind of person has a disease, than what kind of disease a person has.

The purpose of this book is to provide the basic information you, as a health care provider, need in order to know—as Sir Osler suggests—*the kind of people who have health problems.* This book lays the foundation for you to build your own deeper understanding of and appreciation for patients and clients from a variety of diverse populations and cultures.

TERMS USED IN THIS BOOK

Any book that deals with the vague, often nebulous nature of human culture and ethnicity will necessarily include terms that, themselves, are often confusing or even controversial. Throughout this book we use such terms, so it will be helpful to define and discuss them upfront.

As we've already mentioned, we encourage readers to guard against stereotyping, but because we do generalize about the groups we cover in this book, we need to explain the difference between a *stereotype* and a *generalization*. Generalizations are statements about populations that have some basis in fact, for example, "Americans tend to be monolingual and speak only English." Census data and other studies have shown that U.S. Americans as a group generally only speak one language, compared to Europeans and others, who may speak several languages. But this generalization doesn't predict whether a U.S. American actually does speak more than one language. In fact, many U.S. Americans are bilingual or even multilingual. This generalization can also be a stereotype if one assumes that all U.S. Americans are monolingual and should be treated accordingly. When people use stereotypes, they tend to ignore or disregard facts or statements that challenge or reinforce their assumptions about people (Lanier and Davis 2004).

We use the terms *Hispanic* and *Latino* interchangeably in *Health Matters*. Neither term is precise. In general, the United States Census Bureau uses *Hispanic* to classify people "whose origins are from Spain, the Spanish-speaking countries of Central or South America, the Caribbean, or those identifying themselves generally as Spanish, Spanish-American, and so forth. Origin can be viewed as ancestry, nationality, or country of birth of the person or person's parents or ancestors prior to their arrival in the United States." *Latino* is a more inclusive term that covers Hispanics and people with origins in Latin American countries, including Brazil, which is Portuguese speaking.

We discourage usage of the term *race* and promote the term *ethnicity*. *Race* is often used to describe physical differences among people in terms of skin color, hair, or facial features. Most social scientists do not believe that significant physical differences among humans exist. Rather, race is a cultural concept, not a scientific one. Physical differences themselves are meaningless unless people attach meanings to them. *Racism* is the use of negative stereotypes about groups of people or individuals based on perceived physical characteristics.

An ethnic group is a group of people who share a common language, culture, and social views. *Ethnicity* does not rely on the physical characteristics of people. It is closely related to culture, but it is a more precise term that has to do with how people develop a sense of identity as individuals and members of groups. Like culture, ethnicity is flexible, often changing for different situations and through life. A person with black skin might identify himself or herself as Somali or Sudanese and would dislike being called an "African American." Likewise, not all people with light colored skin like to be called "white," perhaps preferring to think of themselves as Italian or Jewish or Irish. The danger in relying on physical characteristics to categorize people is that it contributes to stereotypes. Thinking in terms of ethnicity is more appropriate because it reflects how people understand their own identity, rather than using their appearance to impose an artificial identity on them.

Any detailed discussion of diverse cultures and underserved populations involves the terms *immigrant*, r*efugee*, and *minority*. In many cases, these terms overlap. In other cases, there are significant and meaningful distinctions.

Understandably, people often cannot distinguish among these three groups, but the differences are important for economic, social, and legal reasons. Minority populations, for purposes of this guidebook, refer to those groups of U.S. citizens who are distinct ethnically from the dominant European-American or white majority. This includes African Americans, Asian Americans, Native Americans, and Hispanics. These populations are very distinct from each other, and they have different histories. Take Native Americans, for example. There are more than 500 separate Native

American tribes in the United States. They are indigenous to the nation and are most definitely not newcomers, although they clearly are ethnic minorities and U.S. citizens.

African Americans are also ethnic minorities and U.S. citizens. Many can trace their family histories in the United States back to the 1700s, when they were brought as slaves to the New World. Indeed, African Americans generally have longer family histories in the U.S. than those of many whites from Europe who arrived in the U.S. much more recently. Similarly, many Hispanic Americans can trace their families' presence in the United States centuries before the U.S. even existed.

Minorities, then, are U.S. citizens and have been in the country for many generations, even though they are not of European, white descent. They are also quite different from newly arrived immigrants or refugees. For example, African Americans most likely have far more in common culturally with their white neighbors than with newly arrived refugees from Africa.

The refugee category falls under the immigrant umbrella. In other words, all refugees are immigrants, but not all immigrants are refugees. Important legal distinctions exist between these two groups. Refugees were forced to leave their home countries because of war, political persecution, and/or religious or ethnic intolerance. They are officially recognized by the United Nations as being individuals who cannot return to their homeland because of a well-founded fear of persecution. They come to the United States with a special immigration status that gives them automatic admission into the country and eases their reunification with family members. Someone with a refugee status in the U.S. is given a resident alien card ("green card") and the authority to work in this nation, along with short-term financial assistance funded by the U.S. Department of Health and Human Services through private and state agencies. Refugees are "invited" to live in the U.S. to start a new life.

Immigrants, on the other hand, generally come to the United States for one of two reasons: they are joining family members who already live in this country, or they are "economic migrants" seeking work and better lives for themselves and their families.

Immigrants and refugees have a good deal in common. For example, they come to the United States seeking the things that established residents like about living here. The U.S. provides job opportunities, schooling for children, safe communities, and inexpensive housing. For both populations, coming to the U.S. presents similar challenges; for example, adjusting to a new culture and language. They are often ethnic minorities who may face open racism or other forms of hostility, regardless of their immigration status. For immigrants and refugees who don't speak English, living in U.S. communities—and dealing with the nation's health care system—can cause a tremendous amount of stress.

For the purposes of economy in this book, we use the term *minority populations* for all three groups—minorities, immigrants, and refugees—unless we wish to direct your attention to a specific group. Also, given the wide range of caring professionals who will use this book, we use the terms *patient* and *client* interchangeably.

Finally, a note about how we chose the cultural groups presented in this guide. All groups fit into one or more of the following categories. Some represent the largest minority populations in the United States, including Hispanics and African Americans. Some—namely Latinos and Asian Americans—also represent the fastest growing populations in our society. We also included some of the more recent significant refugee groups. In the 1970s and 1980s, for example, most refugees entering the U.S. came from Vietnam and other Southeast Asian nations. But more recently, in the 1990s and early part of the twenty-first century, refugees have been more likely to arrive from Africa, the Balkans, and the former Soviet Union. Of course, the changing sources of immigrants and refugees not only reflect changes in the locations of major conflict in the world, but it also clearly reflects the globalized nature of the world's economy, in which geopolitical borders have become increasingly meaningless. Finally, we include some minority populations who are particularly unique and pose particularly interesting challenges to health care and social service providers, including Jews (especially Orthodox), the Amish, and Arab Muslims.

PART 1

The Immigrant, Refugee, and Minority Health Care Experience in the United States

AMERICA'S CHANGING ETHNIC LANDSCAPE

The United States is becoming more ethnically diverse. Not only are the nation's established minorities growing rapidly, but immigrants and refugees make up a significant part of the country's population growth. The nation's white population continues to grow, but at a much slower rate than that of minorities. According to U.S. Census Bureau 2000 data, the U.S. white population grew by only 12 percent between 1980 and 2000, while the nation's Asian and Pacific Islander population grew by 204 percent and the Hispanic population grew by 142 percent. During the same period, the nation's black population grew by 31 percent. In other words, between 1980 and 2000, U.S. minority populations grew 11 times faster than the white, non-Hispanic population.

The result of these population trends is that while in 1900 one in eight U.S. Americans was a minority, in 2000, one in four U.S. Americans was a minority. By the year 2050, demographers predict that this figure will increase to more than 50 percent, with no single group representing a majority population anymore. This trend is already occurring in many larger states. Indeed, three states—California, Hawaii, and New Mexico—and the District of Columbia had "majority minority" populations in the 2000 census. Texas was very close, with 48 percent of that state's population composed of minorities. Even small, predominately rural, white states are following this trend and becoming more ethnically diverse, although this is happening at slower rates than larger states with large cities.

Hispanics are the largest minority population in the United States, representing 14 percent of the nation's total population in 2002, or over 37 million people. African Americans represent 13 percent of the U.S. population, or 36 million. The nation's fastest growing minority population—Asians and Pacific Islanders—made up 4 percent of the U.S. population in 2002 (U.S. Census Bureau 2003).

Immigration contributes significantly to the nation's rapid growth in some minority populations. For example, the United States Census Bureau estimated that in 2002 67 percent of the nation's Hispanic population growth was of Mexican origin and that two in every five Hispanic persons were born in another country.

For many states and communities, the arrival and accommodation of immigrant and refugee newcomers, as well as the ability to work with the growing ranks of existing minorities, is critical to their long-term social and economic health. The growth in these populations can bring challenges to health care providers.

CHALLENGES FOR HEALTH CARE PROVIDERS AND MINORITIES, IMMIGRANTS, AND REFUGEES

Serving the health care needs of minorities, immigrants, and refugees can present special challenges for health care providers. In general, by comparison to the white majority population, minorities are disproportionately affected by chronic illnesses, infectious diseases, mental health challenges, accidents, intentional injuries, and other conditions. Interestingly, only a small portion of this disparity is considered to be a result of genetic differences that cannot be changed, such as higher rates of sickle-cell anemia among African Americans and Indians from the Asian subcontinent. More typically, broad differences in income, education, living conditions, lifestyle practices, insurance coverage, family support systems, and other socioeconomic factors have far greater impact on the health status of these groups than do inherent biological differences.

Insurance, Poverty, and Access to Care

Access to care is among the greatest barriers to good health for minorities and newcomers in the United States. Of particular importance is the lack of medical insurance. Minorities are disproportionately represented among the uninsured. In 2003, the U.S. Census Bureau estimated that 20 percent of black Americans and 19 percent of Asian Americans were uninsured. The uninsured rate among Native Americans was 28 percent in 2003. But the rate among Hispanics was even higher at 32 percent—nearly three times the rate of 11 percent among non-Hispanic whites. The large percentage of Hispanics without health insurance may be explained in part by the growing number of Latino immigrants who are in the U.S. without the proper legal documentation and therefore are also unlikely to be uninsured. Indeed, the percentage of the nation's total foreign-born population without health insurance in 2003 was 35 percent, two-and-one-half times that of the population born in the United States, the so-called "native" population (13 percent).

In 2003, the United States Census Bureau also reported that minorities, immigrants, and refugees are much more likely than whites to live in poverty. The poverty rate among the nation's non-Hispanic white population was 8 percent, and the poverty rate among Asians in the same year was 12 percent. Poverty rates among Native Americans, blacks, and Hispanics were significantly higher. Among people who reported themselves as Native Americans of a single indigenous race, rather than mixed with other races, the U.S. Census Bureau indicated that 23 percent lived in poverty. The rate was also 23 percent among Hispanics, and among blacks the poverty rate was 24 percent. Poverty is also higher among the foreign born than natives. Among all people born in the U.S., the poverty rate in 2003 was 12 percent. However, among all foreign-born noncitizens, the poverty rate was nearly twice as high: 22 percent.

Lack of insurance and poverty aren't the only barriers to care for minorities. Geographic restraints are also significant. Health services aren't always located conveniently in ethnic neighborhoods where minority and immigrant populations often live, and they may not have easy car or bus transportation to medical facilities in white areas. Likewise, health services that are only offered from 9:00 A.M to 5:00 P.M., Monday through Friday, off-site in a building staffed by all white providers would typically not be well utilized by many minorities. Many immigrant workers in meatpacking plants, for instance, work double shifts with only one day off per week. They have difficulty seeking care when needed during standard operating hours for most doctors' offices, especially if faced with the added burden of either bringing their children with them or finding suitable childcare.

Cultural access is also a common barrier to care when minority patients cannot be seen by providers familiar with their unique ethnic background or sensitive to their needs. They also may have different health beliefs, attitudes, knowledge, and practices than the white, northern European-descent majority population (see the section "Conceptions of Health" later in this part). In general, because of these and other significant barriers to care, minority patients often seek treatment for health problems later than the majority white population, and they are more likely to present with multiple, more advanced conditions.

Language Barriers

Language issues can also complicate a diagnosis when a patient speaks limited or no English and interpreters aren't available. Sometimes newcomer children have learned some English and are used to interpret in health care settings, but they often lack the English vocabulary necessary to help physicians make accurate diagnoses. The lack of precise interpretation can result in patients' questions not being adequately communicated and doctors' instructions being misunderstood. Many health education programs are developed primarily for white, middle-class populations, and are not culturally sensitive to the specific health practices, needs, and beliefs of minorities.

The Lack of Medical Records

Unlike U.S.-born minorities, refugees and some immigrants often arrive in this country with limited or no health records. Without this background information, it is difficult—if not impossible—for providers to make a fully informed medical diagnosis or even prescribe the best medicine. Lack of medical records can be a very frustrating aspect of working with newcomers for other health care professionals as well. Community health providers, nurses, and others find it impossible to tell if newcomers are allergic to any medications, or if schoolchildren have already received immunizations (perhaps even multiple times) because their shot records haven't been transferred from their native country or refugee camps to U.S. school districts.

New Diseases

Immigrants and refugees can have medical needs that an established community might never have experienced before, like bilharzias (also called schistosomiasis), which is caused by a parasite that invades the urinary system and is common in Africa. Sometimes they bring health problems with them from their home regions, or they might develop the so-called diseases of the poor during their travels. Some of these diseases are also common even in U.S.-born, low-income communities, like tuberculosis. There are also other diseases associated with mobile populations and displacement. In mobile populations, sexually transmitted diseases can be more common, for instance, or prenatal care might have been more limited in native countries or refugee camps.

Conceptions of Health

Different cultures might also have different ideas about what *health* is. For most U.S. Americans, being healthy is the state of feeling well enough to maintain day-to-day activities; a lack of health can be anything that prevents functioning in a normal matter. For immigrants and refugees, being healthy might simply mean a lack of disease. *Unhealthy* could mean that there is disharmony between the body, mind, and spirit because of imbalances and negative energy.

Similarly, ethnic minority and newcomer populations have very different ideas about what constitutes healthy behaviors or what factors cause certain diseases. These beliefs vary dramatically by cultural community. For example, standard U.S. dietary recommendations promote consistent consumption of certain foods, such as dairy products and fresh vegetables, to maintain long-term health. In other cultures, these same foods might be uncommon or only consumed when they are in season.

Differences in what is considered *wellness* can also prevent the U.S. health care system from working adequately for newcomers. For example, the person who has a chronic disease but is still able to function by working and attending to family matters might consider himself "well" and thus not seek medical attention that established residents would consider mandatory. There might also be critical differences in assumptions about how to treat or prevent the condition, and cultural differences can increase the likelihood of a missed or inappropriate diagnosis. The results can be costly if health problems aren't handled appropriately and then become critical and require a visit to the emergency room.

People can also have different ideas about the role of preventive care and health care professionals. Most U.S. Americans understand the importance of preventive and primary health care and the need to establish long-term relationships with physicians. People from countries that lack resources to provide preventive and primary care might consider resorting to doctors only in extreme cases. Many non-Western cultures in the United States have highly developed systems of traditional medicine and healers on which they rely for their main care.

An Intimidating Health Care System

The often impersonal, institutional system of delivering health care common in the United States doesn't always work well with minority and newcomer populations. Many find the typical U.S. health setting socially sterile. This is particularly true for non-Western cultures that are highly focused on the family and interpersonal relationships for healing, and aren't used to external, institutional health care that emphasizes curative treatment rather than the promotion of the patient's holistic well-being. The U.S. health care system is often intimidating to newcomers, and it assumes a level of trust in hospitals, clinics, and doctors that not all minorities, immigrants, or refugees have.

Experience has shown that newcomers are much more likely to use health care programs that reach out to them in a more personal manner. Advertising the availability of special programs for newcomers doesn't often work as well as making personal contact. Making these connections may take time and patience, and might involve identifying and working with leaders in newcomer communities to give outreach programs a degree of legitimacy.

PART 2

Culturally Appropriate Health Care

Providing culturally appropriate health care means that a provider or organization is sensitive to the cultural differences among patients, understands the influence of these differences on their health status, and can modify programs from a practical stand-point to meet the specific needs of diverse clients. Culturally competent health care is necessary because many public health studies around the world consistently indicate that culture is a significant, common barrier to care for minority patients.

Cultural barriers may be quite obvious or more subtle. For instance, a Latino immigrant senior patient may be less likely to visit a local clinic if he knows that the providers there don't speak Spanish, his only language. Likewise, a Somali refugee elder may be reluctant to be seen by a male American physician, because it is disrespectful for her to disrobe in front of a man. Health providers and their agencies, therefore, must be sensitive to the cultural nuances that affect the health status of their minority, immigrant, and refugee patients.

DEFINING CULTURE

The word *culture* is used by many people to mean a variety of things. Phrases such as *workplace culture* or the *culture of an organization* are common. In any human community, culture can be thought of as the "software" in people's brains that determines their behavior, attitudes, basis for distinguishing right from wrong, faith in God, dress, food, and other habits of daily life. Culture is a set of similar ideas and practices shared by a group of people about appropriate behaviors and values. People who share these basic cultural attributes tend to act, eat, and dress the same way, and, in many respects, think in similar ways about life. People usually don't think about their own culture unless they are confronted with another culture. But one way to think about one's own culture is by asking this simple question: "What are the things I do in my normal life that seem so natural that I forget them?" These things make up culture.

Culture is passed from generation to generation, remaining stable over time and shared by everyone in a community. Just the same, culture is also flexible. Cultures share ideas and values with one another, just as people do. A community can thus change its values and behaviors to better meet a changing environment, or because it is exposed to new and better ways of doing things.

CATEGORIZING CULTURE GROUPS

We emphasized the flexible nature of culture and ethnicity in the previous section. Indeed, fitting the world's diverse cultures into a handful of categories is difficult. But we have also found it very helpful for health care professionals and others to categorize types of cultures to help them better understand how cultures differ from one another, and how members of these cultures bring unique perspectives to health care and social service settings.

Categorizing cultures also helps us determine which differences among cultures really make a difference—and which don't. Indeed, most health care practitioners must first learn which cultural category they belong to (become self-aware) before they can begin to understand and appreciate their patients' and clients' cultures.

For several decades, scientists, anthropologists, and others have attempted many schemes to categorize humans. They have used such factors as religion, physical characteristics or *race*, and geography. The problem with using these kinds of factors is that they don't cross-categorize well and they present many inconsistencies. For example, if all Jewish people are categorized as white, this leaves out the ethnic differences between European and Sephardic Jews from Northern Africa and the Middle East. Categorizing Jews as white also leaves out the black Jewish communities in Ethiopia.

We have found Richard D. Lewis' classification categories for cultures the most useful in explaining cultures to our clients (Lewis 2002). Lewis provides three categories of cultures: Linear-Active, Multi-Active, and Reactive. The following lists describe the essential characteristics of these three classifications and the major cultural groups that belong to each.

Linear-Active Cultures
- Value facts and figures
- Respect highly organized planners
- Think linearly
- Use a straightforward, direct communication style
- Take task-oriented approaches
- Prefer rationalism and science over religion
- Typical example cultures include white mainstream Americans and Western Europeans

Multi-Active Cultures
- Value emotions, close relationships, compassion, warmth, and feelings
- Act more impulsively than people from Linear-Active or Reactive cultures
- Prefer face-to-face interaction
- Use direct and animated communication style
- Feel uncomfortable with silence
- Typical example cultures: African Americans, Africans, Arabs, Jews, and Latinos

Reactive Cultures
- Value subtle communication: listen first, then respond
- Honor harmony, humility, and agreement
- Use indirect communication style
- Tolerate silence and find it meaningful
- Typical example cultures: Asian Americans, Pacific Islanders, and Native Americans

CULTURAL COMMUNICATION STYLES

Humans communicate in a variety of ways, both through verbal and nonverbal methods. As you can see in Lewis' cultural categories, people in specific cultures tend to communicate in a similar manner that differs from communication styles in other kinds of cultures. Although any one individual from a certain culture may actually communicate in his or her own unique way, general tendencies within cultures do exist.

For example, the individuals in Multi-Active cultures tend to communicate in an expressive manner. They usually openly display more passion, gestures, and emotion in their communication and may speak more loudly than quieter cultures. They may also stand closer to one another while speaking, or they may touch each other more frequently as a sign of warmth. Language may be very direct and open, with frequent eye contact with each other.

On the other hand, individuals in Reactive cultures are more reserved. Their communication style is more proper, formal, and refined, and may follow specific cultural protocols. Their voice levels are usually lower and their body spacing is greater than in other cultures. Direct eye contact may be avoided, and touch may be less frequent than in other cultures. It may not be proper to ask direct or pointed questions.

For instance, as members of a Linear-Active culture, white U.S. Americans tend to be more reserved than African Americans, but more open than Asian cultures.

To the best of their ability, health providers should be sensitive to and try to adapt to the cultural communication style of their patients. For instance, if patients come from quieter, more reserved cultures, providers must learn to understand and follow the proper protocols of respect in that society. On the other hand, minority patients from more expressive cultures will typically expect closer, warmer, and more trusting relationships with their providers.

PART 3

Becoming More Culturally Appropriate: General Strategies

Most providers have had relatively little meaningful exposure to people from other backgrounds and therefore need to learn how to become more culturally appropriate. Learning these skills, though, can take years of immersion in a particular culture. Furthermore, a provider can be culturally competent with one particular ethnicity of patients but lack experience with other minority populations. Ultimately, becoming competent in this field requires a deep knowledge of the cultural nuances of various groups and an understanding of the unique demographic and socioeconomic factors affecting those populations. Being genuinely friendly, compassionate, respectful, and humble can also go a long way toward making you more culturally competent, even if a provider is unfamiliar with the particular characteristics of a specific group.

GUIDELINES FOR PROVIDERS

As a health care provider who is truly committed to your patients, you should always strive to be as culturally competent as possible with your minority clients, but you also need to keep in mind that culture is only one of many factors that influence the health status of a patient. Age, gender, income, literacy, educational background, lifestyle, amount of time in the United States, individual personality, and so on are equally important factors when you try to gain a complete understanding of a patient. In general, you can follow certain fundamental practices when trying to become more culturally sensitive, regardless of what ethnic group you may be serving.

- Be aware of, and sensitive to, your own cultural values and beliefs as a provider, and recognize how they influence your attitudes and behaviors.

- Be aware of, and sensitive to, the cultural values and beliefs of patients and how they may influence clients' attitudes and behaviors.

- Learn about basic historical events that have affected particular ethnic groups, and understand how oppression, discrimination, and stereotyping currently affect your patients, both professionally and personally.

- Become familiar with your minority clients' traditional health practices, attitudes, and perceptions about various conditions (refer to the culture-specific information in Part 4).

- Determine what communication styles are most common within your patients' particular cultures, and try to emulate them so that your patients relate better to you (see Part 2 for a discussion of communication styles). For instance, some cultures value a more direct, open style of communication, while others tend to be more verbally passive and indirect. Cultures that are more passive may not openly share as much health information with you, so you may need to probe gently with open-ended questions to ascertain a patient's condition.

- Try to be aware of specific cultural "taboos" that apply to a particular ethnic group with which you may be working. For instance, most Jews and Muslims shouldn't be encouraged to follow diets that include pork (see Part 4 for a more comprehensive list of these taboos).

- Make an effort to learn at least a few introductory phrases in their language if you work with patients who don't speak English as their native language; for example, *hello*, *good-bye*, *how are you*, *thank you*, and *please.* This simple act can go a long way toward establishing a friendly and trusting rapport.

- Take the time to ask a lot of questions of your clients—and *listen actively.* Try to treat the *entire patient* in a holistic manner rather than just focus on a particular disease. Learn about the culturally specific risk factors, signs, symptoms, barriers to prevention, and methods of treatment that relate to medical conditions affecting minority patients (see Part 4).

- Learn more about the various cultural communities in your area through (1) interacting informally with individuals from these groups; (2) actively listening to their stories, even if they aren't health related, to learn how their cultural backgrounds impact their experiences in American society; (3) participating in cultural diversity workshops and cross-cultural community events; (4) reading articles and books on cultural dynamics (see Part 5 for a list of suggested readings); and (5) consulting with cultural advisors in your community as situations arise.

- Be humble, genuine, and willing to learn. Know that you will often make mistakes. Don't be afraid to apologize and ask why you may have offended someone. Most individuals around the world, no matter what their ethnic background, will respond positively to sincere, kind, and respectful behavior from others, regardless of whether a particular "cultural taboo" was broken.

- Use a sense of humor. Despite differences in communication styles among cultures, all cultures promote laughter. Humor can go a long way toward breaking down communication barriers and making the provider-patient interaction less intimidating. One particularly helpful trick is to learn a few humorous phrases or words in the patient's language that providers can use to poke fun at themselves. For example, learn a word or phrase that others use to describe people who cannot speak their language. Using such terms not only tells your clients that you can't speak their language, but it often surprises and amuses them as well. It is also very helpful to learn the sentence, "I am learning your language, but I am very slow!"

MAKING HEALTH ORGANIZATIONS MORE ACCOMMODATING

Just as there are multiple strategies that individual health providers can undertake, health organizations can also adopt a variety of deliberate strategies to become more culturally effective with minority patients. (Remember, we are using the term *minority* to refer to immigrants and refugees as well, except where we address one group specifically.) These approaches include the following:

- Health agencies can work together with other organizations in their local community to help provide a welcoming environment for refugees and immigrants. Hospitals and clinics can join schools, law enforcement personnel, social service agencies, houses of worship, libraries, adult education providers, housing authorities, city councils, and the like in sponsoring town hall meetings, diversity information sessions, and other such services to help prepare local residents for any impending arrival of significant numbers of refugees and immigrants to a community. This welcoming environment should also include outreach services for existing minority populations in the community.

- To reduce linguistic barriers to care, health programs should be conducted in the native language of the minority clients that are being targeted for service. Interpreters who are native speakers of the foreign language are usually preferable to those who just speak it as a second language.

- If you work for a health care agency, staff your facility with at least some personnel who are members of the same ethnic minority groups as the patients to reduce subtle cultural barriers to care. These multicultural staff members should be spread throughout your agency or hospital as integral workers and not function merely as interpreters. These employees should work in the front office, support services, and health care provider departments in your agency.

- As often as possible, deliver health care services on-site where minority populations live, work, study, play, worship, shop, and celebrate. Most minority groups in the United States significantly underutilize health care services; therefore, programs that can be delivered on-site tend to be much more effective. Consider conducting screenings, vaccinations, and preventive education programs, for example, in schools, immigrant trailer parks, housing developments, church lobbies, laundromats, ethnic markets, and festival sites for increased access.

- Provide health care services at nontraditional hours. Many minority patients are lower-income and work multiple jobs. Medical offices that are only open weekdays during typical work hours are likely to miss serving large numbers of minority clients. Consider having flexible scheduling on weekends and on at least one or two evenings each week.

- Allow extra time for patient visits when working with refugee and immigrant clients. Many of these people come from non-Western backgrounds that place greater emphasis on face-to-face interaction and don't appreciate being rushed through a medical visit. Many of these clients will present with multiple conditions as well, and will require more than a standard, short visit for care.

- Many non-Western cultural populations place less emphasis on a strict sense of time than mainstream U.S. Americans do.

Appointments and scheduling may need to be flexible when dealing with refugee and immigrant patients in particular, who may not necessarily be willing or able to show up at an exact time on a precise day for care.

• Recruit minority members to serve actively on hospital boards, nonprofit advisory councils, and other external decision-making entities. If they cannot be active on such boards, at least have cultural interpreters in the local community periodically review programs, written material, and policies developed by the health agency for cultural appropriateness.

• Provide extra assistance to refugee and immigrant patients who may have a limited understanding of the complexities of receiving health care in the United States. Many newcomers, for example, are from countries with excellent national health care systems, and they aren't used to having to pay for services, utilize insurance, or fill out claim and aid forms.

• If your clients are very diverse, make sure that signs in your facility are posted in multiple languages. Also, have written health education material and payment forms available in the native languages of your clients. When distributing written material with illustrations, make sure that all photographs or drawings are culturally appropriate.

• Require all staff in your facility to participate in periodic diversity and intercultural training and refresher workshops. Remember that most patients from non-Western cultures place a great deal of emphasis on the word-of-mouth reputation of your health care organization or office. They will care less about fancy marketing brochures than they will about what other minorities say about a particular doctor, hospital, or agency. Make sure that all staff members, including your front office workers, are trained in how to work effectively with immigrant clients to ensure making their experience more positive.

• Draw upon the immense amount of data, studies, brochures, materials, and other sources of information on minority, immigrant, and refugee services that already exist from public health organizations in large urban and border states as well as from federal and international sources. Too often, provider agencies in small rural states feel overwhelmed by the health issues of these groups and often think they must create culturally appropriate programs on their own. Many other states and counties have been actively addressing these health issues for decades and have a wealth of experience and resources to share (refer to Part 5 for information on resources).

PUBLIC HEALTH PLANNING FOR NEWCOMER POPULATIONS

Local public health and social service agencies are often charged with trying to plan short- and long-range services for communities in their district who may be facing influxes of large numbers of refugees and immigrants. Many health agencies often feel drained and overwhelmed when trying to determine what their health priorities should be for these newcomers. However, extensive public health research around the world indicates that these medical concerns are fairly predictable and follow general patterns. If you are a public health planner, you should be aware of the health priorities for intervention that are typically needed by newcomer populations and their host communities. When a refugee group first arrives in your community, you should undertake public health interventions as follows:

• Conduct a rapid public health assessment as soon as possible to determine the general demographics of the newcomer population. This should include getting a general estimate of the total number of new arrivals as well as the general breakdown of people by age groups—such as infants, young children, youths, teens, young adults, middle-aged adults, and seniors—and by gender.

- Assess the overall health condition of the population with any incoming medical records or rapid health assessments of the group's overall condition to determine what existing medical conditions are most prevalent. Of course, it is also important to know the socioeconomic background of the newcomers, such as their general literacy level, reason for arrival, economic history in their former country, and so on.

- Control any infectious diseases (such as tuberculosis) that may be brought in by newcomer populations arriving directly from refugee camps or poor countries. This is necessary both for the immediate health of the newcomers and for protecting the well-being of the host community.

- Triage your population of newcomers into high, medium, and low priority for health interventions. Usually, pregnant and lactating women, young children, the handicapped, and the elderly are at the highest risk initially.

- Work collaboratively with other agencies to ensure that you are adequately meeting the immediate needs of newcomers in areas such as housing and food. Work closely with the city council, churches, schools, law enforcement, and other organizations to address some of these needs and to help prepare the community prior to the arrival of the newcomers.

After the immediate needs of newcomers have been met, shift your public health activities to include the following:

- Conduct public health interventions to address any negative lifestyle practices that will contribute to future chronic diseases. For instance, many immigrants arrive in the United States with better dietary and exercise patterns than those of local residents. These positive practices should be promoted and maintained. All too often, as immigrants and refugees acculturate, they become more sedentary, eat more processed food, and decrease their consumption of fresh produce. Diabetes is one of the most common chronic diseases that develops in immigrant and refugee populations as they acculturate. Also, many immigrant groups arrive with smoking rates that are much higher than those found in the general population, so tobacco reduction programs would be appropriate.

- Implement programs to reduce unintentional injuries and promote safety. Many newcomers work in low-paying jobs (e.g., cleaning houses and hotel rooms) and even dangerous industries (e.g., meatpacking and assembly-line work) that have high rates of accidents. Others may not be aware of U.S. laws requiring car seats for children or smoke detectors in apartments and will need educational programs and consumer health training.

- Provide coordinated, culturally appropriate mental health programs and early intervention projects. Some immigrant and most refugee populations experience some level of mental health challenges. These health problems will vary greatly by individual, age, and gender, as well as by the reasons that caused their immigration or refugee status to occur. For instance, voluntary economic immigrants usually suffer less from depression than refugees, who were involuntarily forced to migrate due to political persecution or war. Also, many of the elderly refugees and immigrants have more difficulty than younger people in acculturating. Many immigrant and refugee parents often experience stress dealing with their children, as traditional social roles change dramatically with acculturation. Likewise, many newcomer men come from cultures where male verbalization of feelings may not be acceptable, or where mental health conditions carry a negative stigma. In general, it is normal for many newcomers to experience some levels of anxiety, depression, acculturation stress, and even post-traumatic stress disorder for at least some time. Some conditions can linger for years if not addressed properly. Family reunification is often the single most important factor that can improve mental health status.

• Implement dental health assessments and treatment programs. Although many newcomers come from countries that have excellent national health care systems, most had relatively little access to good dental care. Newcomers will need dental health assessments and access to primary dental care. Providers should expect to see significant numbers of fairly complicated cases and untreated conditions.

WORKING EFFECTIVELY WITH INTERPRETERS

Many health providers today are finding that they must increasingly work with interpreters to provide their services to immigrants, refugees, and some minority populations. Even if you aren't familiar with a specific ethnic minority population, it is helpful to be at least minimally competent at working with interpreters, which is a skill that you can learn and practice. (*Interpretation* is conversion of spoken or verbal language; translation is conversion of written language.) All too often, for example, a clinician may explain lengthy, complicated directions on how to take medication, only to find that the interpreter summarizes the comments into just a few words. At the same time, many minority patients want to have detailed discussions with their providers about their conditions, but find that the clinicians aren't using the interpreters effectively to solicit this information from them. Health facilities should employ interpreters and train their staff to work effectively with them. The following are general guidelines for utilizing interpreters in a culturally competent manner:

- Speak just a sentence or two, and then stop to let the interpreter convey your statement. Avoid the very common mistake of explaining a lot of information in English, and then waiting for the interpreter to relay your thoughts to the patient. Usually this will result in a large amount of missed information.

- Avoid asking questions that can be answered with a simple *yes* or *no*. The patient may say she or he understands out of fear, concern about losing face, or not wanting to appear uneducated. Ask lots of questions that begin with *why*, *what*, *where*, and *how*.

- Remember to speak to the patient, not the interpreter. The patient should be the focus of your attention. The interpreter merely acts as your voice in the second language. Maintain eye and body contact, if appropriate, with the patient rather than with the interpreter.

- Validate the information that your patient receives from the interpreter. Ask the patient to explain back to you, through the interpreter, whatever information has been shared. This is called *back interpretation*. Ask frequent questions to confirm understanding. For instance, a doctor may ask the client to repeat the prescription instructions he has just given, and a health educator may ask a senior refugee to demonstrate the technique she has just learned for injecting herself with insulin.

- Be sure to use expression and passion in your presentation if appropriate in a health education talk with patients, even if they don't understand your words. Encourage the interpreter to also use the same expression in her presentation.

- Try to make at least some "small talk" with the patients, particularly at the beginning and end of each visit, regardless of the interpreter's presence. Most will understand *hello*, *thank you*, and so on in English. Likewise, as we mentioned earlier, you should learn a few basic friendly phrases or words to share with your clients in their native languages. Smiles, respectful behavior, and a friendly attitude by providers will carry over in any language.

- Speak slowly and carefully in English when working with interpreters. Use simple, plain English, and avoid slang, idiomatic speech, fancy medical terminology, and other types of speech that can easily be confusing for clients and interpreters alike. Expressions like *an arm and a leg*, *cold feet*, and *cough it up* don't interpret well, especially in health care settings!

- Repeat key words, phrases, and medical instructions frequently to ensure that your patients understand them. If not, try to explain the information in a simpler, more practical way. Don't speak loudly as if they are deaf or stupid; they are not. More than likely, the fault will be yours; you are probably not explaining things carefully.

- Rely heavily on demonstrations, visual aids, and culturally appropriate models when teaching patients or groups who aren't native speakers of English. If you are teaching using models, it's best to use real items instead of replicas. Involve the patients in any demonstrations you're conducting.

- Allow patients adequate time to interpret health information for each other when you are working with larger numbers of patients in an audience format. Always ask simple questions to validate their knowledge.

- Avoid using young children or other family members to interpret whenever possible. Confidential health information is less likely to be shared by the patient to the provider in these cases. Likewise, these informal interpreters may not protect the confidentiality of the patient among other extended family members and friends in the ethnic community. Children who may appear to speak English fairly well may not really understand the nuances or the medical vocabulary.

WORKING WITH LOW-LITERACY PATIENTS

Many refugee, immigrant, and even minority populations in the United States have limited written skills in English. Depending on their backgrounds, they may also be unable to read and write in their native language. This will greatly affect their ability to access health care and to use it effectively. Indeed, literacy is one of the strongest, most direct predictors of health status and poverty. For that reason, some of the most effective public health programs for refugees and immigrants actually incorporate literacy and economic development together with health to provide comprehensive solutions for their well-being. If you are working with low-literacy populations, you should be aware of the following general guidelines. Also, keep in mind that although some of your patients may not be literate, that doesn't mean they cannot learn how to improve their health status.

- Maintain a respectful, nonjudgmental, and confidential approach when working with low literacy patients. Although some may come from cultures where low literacy is the norm, this often has a negative stigma in the United States. Health organizations dealing with many refugee and immigrant patients may want to advertise the availability of literacy and English language classes in the local community for their clients.

- Utilize the patient's native language as much as possible when conducting health visits through interpreters, radio programs, and television broadcasts. Avoid relying heavily on written brochures, pamphlets, and handouts, even if they are in the native language of the patients.

- Incorporate ample opportunities for hands-on, interactive health education in nontraditional ways with low-literacy patients. This can include using tools and methods such as real props, visual aids, art therapy, songs, dances, skits, murals, demonstrations, simulations, role playing, games, poetry, weaving, quilting, storytelling, and the like. Many of these "unusual" methods of teaching a health topic are actually very common in many non-Western cultures, and they are quite culturally appropriate for many groups, depending on other factors like age and gender.

- Provide all information in a clear, logical, step-by-step manner for clients.

- Make sure that all verbal material like foreign-language public service announcements, radio shows, television spots, and the like have been pretested by members of the specific ethnic group you are targeting. Many have not been translated by native speakers and often contain glaring mistakes.

- Do not assume that low-literacy patients will automatically understand all visual information provided to them. Many of these clients are also "visually illiterate" and may have difficulty interpreting the meaning of pictures, posters, illustrated brochures, and the like. These materials should be used as a last resort, and should always be pretested before incorporating them into a health education program.

UNDERSTANDING TRADITIONAL HEALTH PRACTICES

Cultures can have very different views and perceptions about what causes disease and poor health. For example, the West emphasizes viewing illness from a scientifically documented knowledge base and uses research and reason to identify the causes of diseases. In these countries, illness is often attributed to very specific, measurable, and identifiable causes such as viruses, bacteria, exposure to toxins, genetic mutations in DNA, consumption of high-fat foods, and the like. Although this is changing, the biomedical model used in the West for understanding health has traditionally placed most of its focus on disease by treating the physical body. There is generally a distinct separation between the mind and body, and limited emphasis placed on emotional, spiritual, or community well-being. Curing disease often requires invasive or aggressive procedures, such as surgery, shots, internal examinations, or chemically based medications.

However, in many non-Western cultures, a much different and broader understanding exists of the determinants of poor health. In general, most of these cultures view health very holistically. Their primary focus is on maintaining wellness through promoting balance between the body, mind, emotions, and spirit, as well as through positive and harmonious relationships with loved ones, the community, and the environment. Each component of this holistic wellness model is equally important, and illness is believed to occur when one or more of these components are out of balance with the others. For instance, emotional distress can negatively affect physical health, just as a community rejecting sacred laws can result in a chaotic, meaningless living environment that would ultimately affect the health of all in a village.

Many East Asian cultures believe that illnesses are the result of blockages in the *chi* energy, or life force, which is thought to permeate all beings. Native American cultures often view some physical diseases as ultimately being caused by the disharmony created when the traditional family structure collapses under poverty and acculturation. Some African cultures attribute illness to the evil eye, demonic possession, or the influences of negative energy in the spirit world when a cultural taboo has been broken. Many Latino, Indian, and other cultures also believe that illness will result when bodily humors, organs, fluids, temperaments, or compositions are out of balance; they are seen as being either too *hot* or too *cold* and must be rebalanced with the opposite force to regain health.

Thus, the perceived causes of illness in many non-Western cultures can be very diverse and often hard to identify or quantify using Western science. These traditional cultures may also have multiple understandings of illness. They could feel that certain diseases that are easily explained by Western science, such as diabetes, was "imported" by outsiders to indigenous cultures, while other conditions are too complex to be attributed to modern biomedical causes. Because of this diversity in the understanding of disease etiology, you should always take the time to assess the unique health beliefs of patients from special populations with which you work. Thoroughly understanding the traditional health knowledge base of an ethnic population can greatly increase your ability to offer culturally appropriate, comprehensive care to patients.

The World Health Organization estimates that up to 80 percent of the world uses herbal medicine and other forms of traditional healing as their primary form of health care. Most of these traditional health practices have been utilized effectively for hundreds and even thousands of years among many cultures. These healing systems are quite different from those used by Western medicine. Traditional health practices around the world are far too numerous to discuss in a guidebook such as this, and they are usually culturally specific. If you will be working extensively with a particular immigrant or minority group, take the time to listen to your patients carefully, ask many open-ended questions, and do further research into the traditional health practices typically utilized by that population. In general, the following information is helpful to understand when trying to work cross-culturally and be respectful of traditional health systems:

• Take the time to learn the culturally specific risk factors, signs, symptoms, barriers to care, and preferred methods of treatment for the minority populations you'll be working with. Public health studies consistently show that this information varies dramatically by ethnicity and culture (see the section "Health Issues and Barriers to Care" for each culture group in Part 4).

- Recognize that most cultures around the world have had a very long history of understanding health and practicing healing in a very holistic way by combining physical health with mental, emotional, spiritual, environmental, and other levels of well-being. The Chinese and East Indians, for example, have extremely advanced written manuals on herbal medicine, manipulation of the human energy field, and other related topics that are thousands of years old. Today, modern medicine is confirming scientifically what many of these practitioners have known for generations. Many Europeans also practiced traditional forms of healing for centuries, even though much of this knowledge is now lost in the West, particularly in the United States, with the medicalization of health through technology and science that is so common in the twentieth century.

- There are a variety of people who perform traditional healing services in many cultures around the world, including shamans, medicine men, wise women, bonesetters, lay midwives, psychics, and energy healers. Unlike in Western medicine, most of the people are not specialists but, as we said, approach health from a very integrated and holistic perspective. There are also many different modalities of traditional healing that are used by practitioners in these cultures. These can range anywhere from herbal treatments and homeopathic remedies to rebalancing the human energy field and intuitive medicine. Acupuncture and yoga are two well-known forms of energy field manipulation in the West that originated in Eastern countries. No matter what traditional practices are utilized in a culture, try to learn about them and the rationale for their usage. Modern scientific medicine is increasingly confirming that the basis for many of these treatments is sound.

- In many traditional practices, the human body, as well as all natural things, is considered infused with a sacred energy or spirit that is connected to the life force of the universe. This energy vibrates and holds emotions and experiences in an aura; shamans and many traditional healers are believed to be able to feel, see, and sense these vibrations. Poor physical health is usually considered to be the result of an energy field imbalance in a nonphysical layer, which weakens the body and allows disease to set in. Healers of various forms using different modalities will manipulate this energy field, cleanse it, unblock it, and rebalance it to bring wellness to the patient.

- In many traditional views, health is not the absence of disease, but a complete, full sense of harmony and balance between body, mind, soul, the family, the environment, and the universe. All things, both living and nonliving, are usually considered to be one and are highly dependent on each other to maintain a balanced and well state. The human body must, therefore, be well balanced and healthy in order to be properly aligned with all other elements of the universe. (It is interesting to note that this "traditional" understanding of health actually correlates strongly with many of Einstein's modern theories on energy, matter, and light.)

- While Western medicine excels at getting rid of symptoms that have manifested in the physical body, traditional healing typically excels at addressing the root causes of poor health, which may have been caused by emotional or psychological distress.

PART 4

The Cultural Communities

The guidelines provided in the previous parts of this book are general recommendations for you and your organization when working with immigrant, refugee, and minority populations. If followed carefully, they will greatly improve your ability to work more effectively with these patients. However, to truly improve cultural competency, you must gain a further understanding of the specific characteristics that are common in particular ethnic and cultural groups.

The information in this part, therefore, will introduce the fundamentals of working with some of the most significant newcomer and minority populations in the United States. Specific cultural communities are featured, and standard information is provided for each group: their historic background in the U.S., language and religion, family and social structure, older adults, cultural and communication style, health issues and barriers to care, bereavement and serious illness, and traditional health practices. In the section "Cultural and Communication Style," we also classify each culture according to Richard Lewis' categorization scheme described in Part 2.

Use the information in this part as a general guide and as a starting point for learning about the basic culture of a client or patient. All people are ultimately individuals, and this information isn't meant to stereotype any group. Remember, as stated previously, age and culture aren't the only factors that influence patient behavior and health status. In an effort to be culturally competent, don't ignore other fundamental factors that are equally important in affecting your patients' health behaviors, such as gender, education level, and individual personality traits. Ultimately, you must be willing to immerse yourself in working with people of diverse backgrounds over an extended period of time if you truly wish to improve your ability to provide services in a culturally appropriate manner.

AFRICAN AMERICANS

Overview

- African Americans have experienced a unique history as a minority population in the United States, and this experience has profoundly affected their socioeconomic and health status. African Americans were the only major ethnic group that came to the Western Hemisphere against their will, and they comprise one of the largest forced migrations of humans in history. In most cases, they were taken from their homes or were prisoners of African wars; separated from their families; confined in slave dungeons in West Africa; transported in cramped quarters on ships across the Atlantic, where many of them died; and then sold to plantation and business owners in the New World.

- African Americans were generally forced to convert to Christianity from their traditional religions, kept uneducated, and were treated as property for decades in the United States. It was only about 140 years ago that slavery was still legal in parts of the U.S, and it was only several decades ago that blacks in many areas of this country, particularly the south, were completely segregated from whites by law in housing, education, and jobs.

- The historically negative relationship between the dominant population in the United States and the minority African American group has had significant impact on the health status of blacks in this country and their use of services. Segregation, institutional racism, poverty, political disenfranchisement, and other such factors in the past have limited the ability of blacks to achieve equality with whites in health, economic, social, education, and related spheres.

Language and Religion

- Because their families have been in the United States for centuries, most African Americans speak English as their native language. A number of black dialects exist, though, that are unique to urban inner cities or rural southern communities.

- Most African Americans devoutly practice some form of Christianity in the United States. Many, particularly those who migrated from the south, are Baptist. The percentage of black Muslims has also been increasing in the U.S., particularly among younger males. Indeed, there are currently nearly 3.0 million African American Muslims in the U.S., which represent 85 percent of all nonimmigrant Muslims in the nation (Wood 2002).

Family and Social Structure

- The family is the foundation of African American society. The family usually revolves around the mother, her elders and siblings, and her children. Fathers may not necessarily live with the family, particularly if they are lower income and the children were born out of wedlock. In general, families tend to be large and caring. Black women are especially recognized for their strength and nurturing tendencies.

- Although African Americans as a group have lower income levels than most other minority populations in the United States, the African American middle class is expanding rapidly in the country. Black women, in particular, have made great strides, and many have become financially successful, although young black males continue to lag behind as a group.

- Many predominantly black communities are organized into neighborhood associations and are connected with a particular local church. These neighborhood associations are often active socially and politically in the community. Take the time to meet the leaders of these neighborhood associations, talk to their residents, and incorporate them into outreach programming. Many health services for blacks will be utilized heavily if they are provided on-site in church basements, schools, neighborhood centers, and the like.

Older Adults

- Older adults in the African American community are highly respected members of the family, and they often heavily influence decisions made within the extended family.

- Older adults may serve as the primary caretakers for their grandchildren. Providers should recognize this extra "caretaker" responsibility, and be aware that there may be questions and medical issues to be addressed as a result. For instance, elderly women may be responsible for purchasing and preparing food for their young grandchildren, but they may have serious medical or financial problems that limit their ability to do so.

- Most African Americans are much more likely than whites to take care of ill older relatives and friends at home rather than send them to formal providers or nursing homes.

Cultural and Communication Style

- In general, many African Americans are more openly expressive than European Americans. They often display more direct eye contact, closer body spacing, and a higher level of physical touch than many whites. Many black children, though, avoid direct eye contact with adults out of respect.

- Verbally, African Americans may be more likely than whites to share their opinions openly or ask questions directly. They may also display a higher level of verbal emotion and expression than European Americans. When planning health services, you should adjust to these cultural nuances and use interactive activities that allow ample opportunity for discussion, problem solving, and hands-on learning.

- Lewis Culture Category: **Multi-Active**.

Health Issues and Barriers to Care

- Cost is generally the greatest barrier to care for African Americans in the United States.

- Some public health studies have shown that blacks have a low level of trust in the U.S. medical system and its providers, who are primarily white. This mistrust is a very important cultural barrier to care and should not be underestimated. Actively focus on developing trusting, warm, and respectful relationships with your African American patients.

- Many African Americans, even those who are highly successful and educated, feel that the historical legacy of slavery, segregation, unethical scientific experiments, ethnic profiling, and other human rights abuses over the past several centuries have significantly damaged black-white relationships in the United States; it will require additional time and effort to reconcile these issues. As such, many African American patients question the methods and motives used by white providers and health organizations that provide them with care, and blacks will often be particularly sensitive to and insulted by poor treatment from white providers.

- It is important to recognize the implications that the legacy of slavery and discrimination has had on the health status of African Americans. Because it has only been in the last few decades that discrimination has become illegal, a number of factors combine to put African Americans at very high risk for poor health, such as lower income and education levels.

- As a group, the health status of blacks is among the worst in the nation, with significantly higher morbidity and mortality rates for almost all diseases and injuries in comparison to whites and many other minority groups. Some of these figures are due to genetic factors, but most are a result of higher poverty and unemployment levels, lower education and literacy levels, institutional bias based on ethnicity, more single-parent families, limited financial and cultural access to health care, and lifestyle factors.

- Blatant as well as more subtle forms of discrimination likely contribute to higher levels of stress among African Americans, which can negatively affect their health status as it contributes to hypertension, low birth weight, headaches, and other conditions.

- Blacks are disproportionately represented among those on federal or state medical assistance programs, as well as among the unemployed and underemployed.

- African Americans don't always access medical care in a timely, preventive-oriented manner. They often wait to enter the system until their medical conditions have become complicated and pronounced. Early intervention programs are best provided on an outreach basis in schools, neighborhoods, churches, and other locations where African Americans meet, rather than waiting for them to come to clinics for care.

- Hypertension, diabetes, heart disease, cancer, accidents, and violence are among the most commonly reported health conditions affecting blacks. Their burden of disease can be much higher than that for whites, as it relates to death and illness rates for many conditions.

- Stress and depression can be significant mental health challenges among African Americans, and many cite discrimination as a major factor affecting their well-being. Fear of racial profiling, for instance, may cause older black women to be reluctant to leave their neighborhoods and can contribute to feelings of helplessness and fear.

Serious Illness and Bereavement
- Bereavement practices vary somewhat among African Americans and depend on the religion practiced by the patients. In general,

many African Americans, particularly women, are deeply spiritual and place great emphasis on their religious values. The patient's minister or other religious leader should usually be notified in the case of serious illness or death.

• Many extended family members and friends, particularly women, will likely visit patients who are ill or have died. Visitors may be visibly upset about the condition of the patient. In some cases, where the communication between health providers and family members has been poor, visitors may be suspicious about what caused the death or illness of the patient.

• Cremation is less common among African Americans than it is among whites.

• Most African Americans are reluctant to allow organ donations by family members, but will generally allow autopsies when necessary.

Traditional Health Practices

• Public health studies clearly show that African Americans as a whole often have different health beliefs and attitudes about various medical conditions than do whites or other ethnic populations, as discussed in the following bullet points. Take the time to really listen to your patients and try to understand why they may feel a certain way about a condition.

• In general, African Americans have been shown to attribute their health status to factors outside their own control, that is, fate and destiny. In other words, while whites may feel that they can control many things in their own lives, blacks are more likely to feel that factors other than their own behaviors are the cause of various life events. Encouraging African American clients to develop a sense of empowerment and personal involvement with their own health may be helpful.

- God is seen as a source of significant strength in times of illness and poor health. Indeed, many blacks place greater emphasis on the role of God in healing disease than in medical providers.

- Africans, when they were first brought to the United States several centuries ago, carried with them a wealth of knowledge regarding traditional healing through herbs, rituals, and spirituality. Much of this direct knowledge from West Africa was eventually lost over the years, although many continue to value alternative, more natural treatments to care.

THE AMISH

Overview

- The Amish are one of the oldest and most unique minority populations in the United States, with many of them first coming to this country from the region around Switzerland several hundred years ago to avoid religious persecution.

- The Amish practice a traditional form of Christian fundamentalism that has changed little since their settlement in the United States. They are well known for their preference to remain apart, by and large, from mainstream American society so that they may practice their traditional lifestyles. Pennsylvania, Ohio, Iowa, Wisconsin, North Dakota, South Dakota, Kansas, and other rural areas are among the states with the greatest populations of Amish in the U.S.

- There are numerous sects of conservative, traditional Amish. As a group, they generally shun most use of modern technology, as they believe it draws people away from a more natural, simpler lifestyle that is closer to God. Therefore, health programs shouldn't incorporate telephones, driving, electrical equipment, computers, or other such technology when educating the Amish.

Language and Religion

- The Amish are usually not native speakers of English, but rather speak an old dialect of German called *Deitsch*, or Pennsylvania Dutch. You will want to use an Amish interpreter for your work, unless the clients are familiar enough with English.

- The Amish generally follow a very strict interpretation of the Bible and are devout Christians. Health services shouldn't be conducted on Sundays or religious holy days with them. They usually don't celebrate nonreligious holidays like the Fourth of July. Also, human or God-like traits such as faces usually shouldn't be assigned to health education props, like dolls or models.

Family and Social Structure

- The Amish are a rural people with very large families. Most marry young and don't use birth control. It isn't uncommon for Amish women to have seven or more children.

- The Amish generally marry only other Amish, so most are related in some way to other Amish.

- Gender roles are usually strong in Amish culture: men serve as the head of household and are responsible for heavy farming and building duties, while women and children tend to the home and family garden.

Older Adults

- The Amish usually take care of their own elders until they die, and keep them active in the family unit. Many build an addition to their homes so that their aging parents can live with them. Amish families are therefore usually multigenerational.

- Children are expected to act disciplined when around adults; they must obey and honor their elders. Seniors are esteemed for their knowledge and wisdom, and are generally shown great respect and care.

Cultural and Communication Style

- The Amish, in general, are a very stoic, decent, honest, hard working, devout, and respectful group of people. They tend to treat others with these positive traits and expect the same in return.

- The Amish typically don't allow people to take photographs of them. Exceptions, though, are often made in medical necessity situations as they relate to x-rays, CT scans, and the like.

- In general, the Amish maintain a respectful distance and mini-mize touching, particularly between males and females. You should also maintain appropriate body space when working with them and avoid excessive physical contact.

- Dress very modestly when you are working with or treating Amish in order to respect their traditional values. Women should wear long skirts or dresses, with their arms, legs, and chests covered to a large extent. Muted colors are usually most appropriate.

- The Amish typically study in one-room schoolhouses, with all ages and both genders together through eighth grade. After that, they usually return to their farms. Students are usually highly disciplined and respectful to health educators, although potentially shy and passive. Literacy rates among the Amish are usually fairly low, so you'll want to rely more on face-to-face and visual learning.

- Lewis Culture Category: **Reactive**.

Health Issues and Barriers to Care

- Culture is a significant barrier to care for the Amish. They typically don't use Western medicine unless it is absolutely necessary or if an illness is in an advanced state. For instance, most won't get prenatal care until the very end of a term, and most give birth at home after the first child. Many would prefer to avoid or delay getting vaccinations.

- The Amish don't have medical insurance. They pay for their care in cash and not with credit. Large medical bills are usually covered communally through Amish financial cooperatives. Expensive medical procedures shouldn't be ordered for Amish patients unless absolutely necessary.

- As the Amish are rural dwellers, most don't live near any health facilities and thus require transportation for medical care. Many have relationships with non-Amish farmers, or *English* drivers as they are called, who can transport them to medical facilities if needed.

- Maternal and child health, infectious diseases, farm safety, and buggy accidents are among the most common health conditions they face. They are typically quite fit and have low rates of obesity. Because of intermarriage with cousins, some genetic conditions such as Hemophilia B, phenylketonuria, metabolic disorders, deafness, and dwarfism can be seen more frequently among the Amish.

- The Amish view good mental and physical health as a blessing that is the result of God's will, and a direct outcome of hard work, decent behavior, and a proper lifestyle. The Amish generally continue working until they truly are too ill to do so, at which time other Amish community members willingly assist them in their chores.

- Although they generally shun technology, the Amish usually accept medical procedures that are necessary for their health, but you'll need to clearly explain the importance of these technological processes. Also, because they have no electricity at home, they cannot use medical rehabilitation devices such as adjustable mechanical beds, unless they can operate without power.

- In strict interpretation of the Bible, the body is viewed as God's temple, and the person has a responsibility to maintain his or her health. Invasive procedures are generally not preferred unless necessary.

- In keeping with their cultural and communication style, the Amish of all ages tend to be stoic in their expression of pain. They may also be too reserved to disclose intimate, personal health information, particularly as it relates to mental health conditions or sexual disorders.

- Modesty is valued by the Amish culture, so special care should be taken with hospital clothing and medical procedures to maintain the dignity of the patient.

- Because children are viewed as gifts from God, and handicaps are His will, the Amish don't allow abortion or many kinds of prenatal testing.

- Although Amish adults value clean living and shun the use of most addictive substances, Amish teenagers are allowed to experiment with a non-Amish, material lifestyle before deciding if they wish to officially become part of their church community. Therefore, some young Amish do use cigarettes, alcohol, and perhaps other drugs.

Serious Illness and Bereavement

- As devout Christians, the Amish generally believe that life on earth must be lived well and oriented to God so as to enter heaven upon death.

- If possible, the Amish patient should be allowed to die at home instead of in a hospital.

- The Amish don't usually embalm their dead. Instead, they typically bury them shortly after death directly into the ground. In rural areas, special group plots are set aside in the community as graveyards, where several dozen Amish may be buried.

- Amish cemeteries, in keeping with their lifestyle, are plain and simple, and lack ornate decorations, flowers, and detailed descriptions of the dead common in many American cemeteries.

- In general, the Amish are fairly reserved in their expression of grief and mourning. They tend to view death as simply a natural process that will ultimately bring them closer to God.

- The Amish usually work closely as a community to help the single head of household after the death of a spouse. Many come together to help widows, in particular, with plowing, harvesting, and other difficult farm duties.

- As the body is viewed as sacred, organ donations are generally not approved by family members, nor are autopsies unless legally required.

Traditional Health Practices

- The Amish usually feel that God's will determines their health, so public health workers should make appropriate adjustments in their presentations to allow for this strong belief in fate.

- The Amish typically value the use of natural remedies as their first choice of care. Many are reluctant to follow the medical advice of physicians because they prefer less invasive methods of treatment.

- Most Amish also have a great interest in herbal medicine. Many women share medicinal recipes with other Amish, and frequently make their own herbal remedies for their families. They may pick medicinal plants in the rural fields surrounding their farms and then make infusions out of them. Many Amish stores, which are frequently based out of homes, carry a large line of homeopathic medicines and vitamin supplements for other Amish to buy.

- In some cases, the Amish seek out local healers in the community to conduct *Brauche* with them. In this traditional procedure, lay healers place their hands on the Amish patient near important parts of the body (like the head or abdomen) to extract illness from the body.

ARAB MUSLIMS

Overview

- Arab culture exists in many countries around the world that speak Arabic as their primary language. These Arab countries range from those in North Africa, like Tunisia, Egypt, and Morocco; to those in the Eastern Mediterranean and Middle East, like Lebanon, Jordan, and Iraq; and south to those on the Arabian Peninsula, like Oman, Yemen, and Saudi Arabia.

- Arab culture is among the oldest and most advanced in the world. Its rich history of art, philosophy, education, music, literature, and religion is well recognized, and it has influenced other societies around the globe for centuries.

- In the United States today, there are between 1.5 and 3 million Arabs and people of Arab ancestry. Many came to this country initially as migrants seeking greater economic opportunities, or as political and religious dissidents fleeing government establishments in their native countries. More recently, many Arabs are coming to the U.S. as scientific or technology specialists, working in the fields of mathematics, computer science, academia, and others.

Language and Religion

- The language spoken by Arab Muslims is Arabic, although the dialects vary widely from country to country.

- Most Arabs, although not all, practice Islam; people who practice Islam are called Muslims. Islam is one of the world's three great monotheistic religions, along with Judaism and Christianity. Muslims share a belief with Christians and Jews in the Old Testament and in one god (*Allah*), but they also follow the Muslim holy book, the Koran, and the teachings of the prophet Muhammad. Jesus is recognized as a prophet and holy man, but not as a Messiah as in Christianity.

- The Islamic faith came out of Middle Eastern traditions, as did Christianity and Judaism, and is the fastest growing religion on earth. In the United States, much of the rapid growth of Islam can be attributed to African American males. Islam is the state religion in many Arab nations.

- Arab Muslims can range from being secular to very devout. Most are fairly conservative in the practice of their religion.

- Devout Muslims worship at a mosque, not at a church or synagogue. Friday is their holy day of rest and worship. They generally greatly resent any efforts to convert them to Christianity, particularly because of the historical persecution of Muslims by Christians during the Crusades and other events.

- Devout Muslims usually pray five times a day, from the early morning through the evening. They pray in the direction of Mecca, one of the holiest cities in Saudi Arabia, from wherever they are in the world. If Muslim patients are staying in a hospital, all staff should be able to tell them what direction Saudi Arabia would be for them, so that the patients can pray to Mecca (usually east in the U.S).

- Most Muslims practice a month of fasting from sunrise to sunset, called *Ramadan*. This ninth month of the Islamic year varies from the Gregorian calendar year to year. No food, water, medications or smoking are allowed during the day during Ramadan. Devout Muslims don't drink alcohol at any time of the year.

Family and Social Structure
- Devout Arab Muslims usually have well-defined, traditional roles for men and women. Ideally, the sex of the provider should match the sex of the patient when working with devout Muslim clients.

- Arab Muslims usually value large families and greatly adore children. Birth control isn't desired in devout families because of the value placed on children.

- Arab Muslims generally don't practice abortion. Circumcision is performed on all boys, although the timing can vary from birth until puberty. Devout Arab Muslims also recognize Islam's prohibitions against premarital sex and adultery.

- Arab Muslim mothers are greatly revered for their role as keepers of the home and family, and they have important power and influence on these two social institutions that are most valued by the culture. This female role is seen as sacred, powerful, and separate from that of men in traditional Arab culture, and *not necessarily subordinate to males as is portrayed in the West.*

- At the same time, men in this patriarchal culture are recognized as heads of the household, and they play strong decision making and leadership roles for the family in public. Protecting and supporting the family, as well as maintaining its honor, are integral responsibilities of males in Arab Muslim culture.

Older Adults
- Muslim families have an obligation to take care of their elders without institutionalization.

- In general, age is greatly respected in Islamic society, and elders are valued for their role in passing on traditions and cultural heritage. Seniors play powerful roles in decision making in families.

Cultural and Communication Style
- In general, Arab Muslims value a communication style that is warm, honorable, and respectful to others. Although Arab culture has a rich history of literature and the written word, it is

also highly verbal. Conversations are often lively, opinionated, expressive, and animated, with frequent metaphors and parables.

- Arab Muslim society places great value on honor and in maintaining proper appearance in public. Disrespectful behavior will be remembered and greatly resented. Shame is also an important concept in Arab culture, and is used often to promote certain social behaviors and expectations.

- Men and women usually avoid direct eye contact and physical interaction unless they are related, as it can imply sexual desire.

- Body spacing between family members and relatives is usually close and affectionate, with frequent touching. Among friends, it isn't unusual for men to hold and touch each other, and for women to do the same with other females.

- Hospitality and reciprocity are also two cultural traits that are very important in Arab Muslim culture. Arab Muslim families that don't show graciousness, warmth, and generosity to guests and outsiders will often face a shameful reputation in the culture. Likewise, an Arab Muslim who helps another will usually expect that assistance to be repaid in the future through a similar act.

- Lewis Culture Category: **Multi-Active.**

Health Issues and Barriers to Care
- Barriers to care such as transportation, cost, and language generally vary among Muslim clients according to ethnicity, rather than religion, because of the diversity within this group.

- Good health is often viewed as being a blessing from God, and illness can be seen as the result of God's will as well. It can also be attributed to poor diet, limited personal relationships, stress, and the like. Arabs generally feel that being well-fed and warm can help promote good health.

- Arab Muslims generally pay significant respect to educated medical providers like physicians. These patients are usually quite compliant and respectful, particularly if the rationale for a particular procedure is explained well.

- Arab patients may get particularly anxious when alone in the hospital, and most prefer to have a lot of family members and friends visit with them at all hours. Many wish to have some loved ones sleep with them in the hospital.

- Many Arab Muslims recite the Koran near the patient, which they prefer to do discreetly. It is usually inappropriate for them to pray in the chapel room of many hospitals, because there often are Christian crucifixes posted.

- Exposure of body parts of the Arab Muslim patient should be kept to a minimum. Loose hospital gowns that open in the back usually cause great embarrassment to the Arab Muslim patient. Some hospitals are now providing pajama pants for Arab Muslim male and female patients for greater modesty. Most Arab Muslims also don't like to be disrobed with other family members present, unless they are of the same sex. Do not touch the patient's head or hair, unless necessary for an exam, and then explain this to the patient beforehand. Many traditional Arab Muslims, particularly women, wear some sort of head covering, such as a scarf, out of modesty and religious devotion. Don't ask female patients to remove these head coverings unless absolutely necessary. If so, again, be sure to explain why you need to remove the covering.

- Arab Muslims tend to be very expressive and verbal in pain as a way to let family members know how serious their experience is.

Some even fear pain and may be quite anxious before receiving medical treatments. Thorough explanations of the necessity and mechanics of any medical procedure by health providers can reduce this anxiety.

- Mental health issues, particularly among men, aren't always acknowledged in public or to providers because they may be perceived as embarrassing. Arabs may be experiencing depression if they seem unusually sad and don't display much emotion in their conversation or behavior. Professional help is often not sought until the condition is much more advanced. Mental illnesses are sometimes attributed to God's will.

Serious Illness and Bereavement

- Most Arab Muslims believe that life on earth is to be spent preparing for another world after death.

- Many Arab Muslim families prefer that they be informed first by health providers about a grave prognosis for patients, so they can protect the ill from bad news. An elder male is usually the family spokesperson, but many health decisions are made in an egalitarian way with all adult family members.

- In general, Arab Muslims do not embalm. The body is usually washed and purified in a ritual manner, and then covered in a simple *kafan*, or cloth. The deceased is then buried in the ground directly after the funeral. The burial usually takes place fairly quickly after death. Direct burial in the ground is required by *Shariah*, or Islamic law.

- Death is viewed as being predestined by God, and it is just the beginning of eternal life. As such, some very religious Arab Muslims may be quite stoic and calm in their mourning. The outward expression of grief through wailing and banging the chest is forbidden. Grieving is usually allowed for just three days.

- Large numbers of extended family and friends usually visit seriously ill or deceased patients. Mourners join together to offer *janazah* prayers for heavenly compassion and forgiveness for the deceased. An additional janazah prayer is often said upon burial. Meals from home may also be brought to sick patients, especially if a hospital cannot provide the proper food to meet Muslim dietary codes.

- Upon death in a hospital, try to turn the face of the patient so that it faces the direction of Mecca in Saudi Arabia.

- Most Arab Muslims prefer to be buried in cemeteries set aside for followers of Islam.

- Arab Muslims usually do not approve of autopsies or organ donation.

Traditional Health Practices

- Traditional health practices of Arab Muslims vary by ethnicity and country of origin. Most Muslims don't eat pork products, shellfish, or other foods that are deemed unclean and unhygienic. Meat products will only be eaten if they are *halal*, or have been slaughtered according to strict practices. (This is somewhat similar to the kosher dietary rules in Judaism.) Hospital food and diets should be modified to meet their needs. They typically share food, and they are often taught not to eat to capacity. Some food, therefore, may remain untouched. Devout Muslims won't eat any food product made with lard or animal fat, like some ice cream, gelatin, and fried foods. As mentioned earlier, they also don't drink alcohol.

- Arab Muslims generally consider the right hand to be clean, and use it for eating, shaking hands, and touching others. The left hand is considered unclean and is reserved for toileting and other such practices. Providers should minimize touching

Muslim patients with their left hands. Ritual cleanliness of the body and home is usually extremely important to Muslims, particularly during times of prayer.

- After birth, many Muslim parents will take the placenta and dispose of it for burial in accordance with Islamic tradition. Fetuses after the age of 120 days are considered viable babies and require burial by Muslims.

BOSNIAN REFUGEES

Overview

- Many immigrants from the former Yugoslavia, particularly Bosnia, now reside in the United States. Many of them came in the mid-1990s as war refugees, and were granted legal permission by the U.S. government to settle throughout the country. Many of the Bosnians, known as *secondary migrants*, first settled in areas like Utica, New York, where they were recruited to work in manufacturing and other industries. Once in the U.S., many resettled later in other states, like those in the Midwest and beyond, drawn by recruitment efforts from other industries and the preference to live together in defined ethnic communities with relatives.

- Because they are classified as refugees, most Bosnians qualify for a number of special federal and state benefits in the health, business, and human service sectors. They are generally legal residents.

- Be sure to remember that Bosnians, unlike many other Eastern European immigrants, were forced to flee their homeland due to ethnic conflict and didn't come voluntarily to the United States like economic migrants. Many would prefer to be back in Bosnia if the political situation was different, and they generally resent people who think they came to the U.S. looking for work.

- Bosnia is quite well developed and cosmopolitan. These newcomers will resent providers who speak down to them and imply that the Bosnians came from a "backward" country. Many Bosnians were professionals in their home country; in fact, most were doctors, nurses, teachers, and business leaders. Many would like to resume their professions in the United States, particularly as medical providers, and they should be utilized in refugee programming.

Language and Religion

- Bosnia was one of the six republics that made up for the former Yugoslavia, and it was the most ethnically diverse. Most of the Bosnians speak Bosnian, which is similar to Serbo-Croatian, as their first language. Some of the younger Bosnians, and those who were educated professionals back home, arrived in the United States knowing at least some basic English. Others learned second languages such as German, because they may have been housed in transit refugee settlements for several years before receiving permission to come to the U.S.

- While most Bosnians are Muslim, most are fairly secular in their practices. You should be familiar with Muslim practices, but don't assume, for instance, that Bosnian women wear veils and long dresses. Most Bosnians don't eat pork. More information about such practices may be found in this guidebook under the language and religion section for Arab Muslims.

Family and Social Structure

- Within the nuclear family, Bosnian Muslims commonly have two or three children. However, a large extended family comprised of cousins, second cousins, aunts, uncles, and other relatives is greatly valued.

- Many Bosnians also have strong connections with their home-towns and usually readily identify themselves by those communities. Some of these towns fought against each other during the Balkan War, and post-war animosity among ethnic groups can still run strong.

- Within Muslim families, males play important leadership and decision-making roles in public. Women are greatly respected for their roles in leading the daily activities of the family at home.

- Maintaining family honor and avoiding shame and public embarrassment can be important cultural factors that influence Bosnian group and individual behavior.

Older Adults

- Bosnians greatly value extended family ties. Many have now been successful in bringing additional family members, like grandparents, over to the United States.

- Many Bosnian families are multigenerational. Grown children are usually excellent caretakers of their elderly parents and don't like to put them into nursing homes. Likewise, young children usually treat their elders with great respect. Public health programming should therefore target the entire family unit rather than just the individual.

- Working with an interpreter may be important when communicating with the older adult Bosnian population. Many of them have only recently come to the United States and are still learning English, a language they (and many others) often find extremely difficult. Successful health programming with older adults has been done by some organizations using an interpreter, who, for instance, could help conduct educational activities informally with the seniors as they drink Turkish coffee and share sweets with each other in their homes.

Cultural and Communication Style

- Most Bosnians value a warm, open, direct, and respectful form of communication with others. Bosnians are also well known for their sense of humor and positive outlook on life.

- As a Muslim society, traditional social values such as dignity, honor, and respect are integral to Bosnian culture. Reciprocity of hospitality, gifts, and other symbols of the importance of relationships are very important to this population. Failure to show the appropriate level of respect or reciprocity to another can bring shame upon a family.

- Lewis Culture Category: **Multi-Active.**

Health Issues and Barriers to Care

- As true war refugees, many Bosnians have experienced extremely difficult circumstances before arriving in the United States. Many lost their homes and livelihoods, and most have close family members and friends who died in the war. Some were deeply traumatized by ethnic cleansing, war injuries, torture, group rape, and other human rights abuses.

- Significant mental health challenges, such as depression, anxiety, and post-traumatic stress, are common human reactions to uncommon circumstances like ethnic cleansing and forced migration. Health providers should expect to see higher rates of these conditions in Bosnian refugees than in the general population of immigrants. However, because many Bosnians feel that mental health conditions have a negative stigma, they may be reluctant to discuss such conditions with providers. Mental health providers should be trained in the complexities of dealing with war refugees, and clinicians shouldn't push a trauma victim to share feelings or experiences until he or she is ready. Provide gentle, ample, and supportive opportunities for them to do so—and be patient.

- Bosnians generally have high rates of smoking and drinking alcohol, as these are integral cultural practices. They may not be familiar with U.S. laws prohibiting the purchase of alcohol by children for their parents, and they may have some difficulty getting used to the anti-smoking mentality in the United States. Second-hand smoke and prenatal smoking are often issues that need public health intervention as well.

- Modesty, especially among older Bosnians, may prevent them from effectively conducting breast self-examinations and other preventive procedures at home. Some will also be uncomfortable wearing open or loose hospital gowns that expose too much of their bodies to staff and visitors.

Serious Illness and Bereavement

- Large numbers of extended family members and friends will likely come to visit the seriously ill or deceased patient. They often gather to offer special prayers of compassion and forgiveness for the deceased.

- Bosnians typically prefer to be buried in special cemeteries set aside for Muslims.

- Bosnian Muslims believe that life on earth is to be spent preparing for another world after death.

- In general, Bosnians don't embalm. The body is usually washed and purified in a ritual manner and then covered in a simple cloth. The deceased is buried in the ground directly after the funeral. The burial usually takes place fairly quickly after death. Direct burial in the ground is required by *Shariah*, or Islamic law.

- Bosnians also generally do not support autopsies or organ donation.

Traditional Health Practices

- Herbal infusions, alcohol-based tinctures, and other forms of traditional medicine were commonly used in Bosnia for generations, and can still be found as over-the-counter medications in many Bosnian ethnic markets. Be aware that many Bosnians will use these remedies simultaneously with Western medicine. Providers may want to ask their patients about the use of these self-help treatments to avoid any possible contraindications.

- Bosnians practice many of the same traditional health practices as other Eastern Europeans. For more information, refer to the section "Traditional Health Practices" for Russians and Eastern Europeans later in this book.

EAST AFRICAN REFUGEES

Overview

- Africa is the continent most affected by poor health and civil strife in the world, and it significantly lags behind in many public health indicators. Increasingly, Africans are fleeing violent ethnic conflict, severe poverty, and political oppression as refugees, and are being granted asylum in industrialized Western nations like the United States and Canada. In recent years, there has been an influx of East African refugees and immigrants, primarily from Somalia, Ethiopia, Eritrea, and Sudan.

- Most of the Somalis, Ethiopians, Eritreans, and Sudanese came from impoverished settings. Many of them don't have the skills necessary to work in an industrialized country, and often require some form of vocational training before getting jobs in the United States.

Language and Religion

- East African countries, like all of Africa, are far more diverse than the United States, so generalizations are difficult to make. However, most of the Ethiopians and Eritreans speak Afar, Arabic, Amharic, Tigrigna, or Oromigna, while the Somalis typically speak Somali, which had no written script until 1972. The Sudanese may speak Arabic, Nuer, Dinka, or other languages.

- East Africa has some of the lowest literacy rates in the world. For instance, the United Nations Development Program (2003) cites adult literacy rates over the age of 15 that range from only 40 percent in Ethiopia to 59 percent in the Sudan. Because of these low literacy rates and the highly verbal nature of East African culture, focus on conducting programs that are primarily oral and in the native language, and avoid heavy utilization of written information in any language. These patients may find filling out forms and paperwork to be overwhelming and frightening.

- Most of the Ethiopians are Coptic Orthodox Christians, while many Muslims come from Eastern Ethiopia and Eritrea. Most of the Somalis are devout Muslims, so providers should follow guidelines for working with patients from this faith, which can be found in the "Language and Religion" section of the Arab Muslim chapter in this book. Most of the Somalis dress modestly, particularly the women, who often wear loose, long dresses and headwraps.

- Sudan is one of the most diverse countries in the world, and its refugees come from many backgrounds. In general, though, most of the Sudanese refugees come from the south of the country, and are either Christian or practice some form of indigenous spirituality. Many have been persecuted in civil war by Muslims in the north.

Family and Social Structure

- The family is the basis of East African society. The families are extremely large, with many children and extended relatives. They also try to remain living in close proximity to each other as they get older. In the United States, where some have resettled without family members, other African friends play an important social role by providing close companionship, support, and mutual help to each other.

- Children are greatly loved and adored, so birth control and abortion are usually not practiced. Handicaps are believed to be the will of God.

- During the first few years of life, young children tend to be sheltered and protected from the broader world, and they spend a lot of time with their parents. Childcare outside family members and friends is not usually sought. Maternal and child health is a priority public health focus with these newcomers.

- Men are usually considered to be the main providers and protectors for the family, and are expected to remain strong during times of crisis. The women, even if they work outside the home, are the primary caretakers of children, the ill, and the family.

Older Adults

- Young people traditionally showed great respect for their elders, and age is valued in traditional East African societies. Out of deference, titles such as *auntie* and *uncle* are sometimes used with elders, even if they are strangers.

- Elders often play an important role in recommending a course of action if a family member is ill or experiencing conflict. As such, older members of the family can play a valuable part in problem solving. Older women, for instance, are often consulted for advice on childrearing, and may even help actively raise their grandchildren by living with their adult children for a while.

- As a result of the large family network, East Africans normally prefer to take care of their own elders at home. However, because young people are increasingly working outside of the home, this tradition is changing.

Cultural and Communication Style

- East Africans usually are fairly soft spoken, respectful, and reserved. Women and children may be more likely to show some emotion than men. Maintaining dignity and respect with each other is important. They are intensely private people and may be unwilling to share intimate personal information in their early contacts with health providers.

- East Africans usually give a great deal of respect to elders and to people in positions of power, like physicians. They are usually fairly passive and won't ask a lot of questions, even if they don't understand something, because they consider that disrespectful. They may also be reluctant to ask for help.

- Interaction between males and females is generally quite proper and defined, and should be respected. Male providers should generally not shake hands with females. Where possible, male providers should see male clients, and female clinicians should see female clients. Eye and physical contact between men and women is usually avoided in public out of respect. Don't misread such lack of eye contact as avoidance.

- Multiple kisses on each side of the face can be a common greeting among East African families and friends.

- If you visit the homes of East Africans, avoid sitting with the soles of your shoes pointing to them—this can be considered disrespectful, because the soles of one's shoes are considered unclean. Also, don't motion for them to come with your index finger, as that signal is reserved for communicating with animals.

- Many immigrants from East Africa have different concepts of time than that in the West. It isn't uncommon for them to miss medical appointments and come at completely different times. They also usually won't call to cancel. Rather than force them to fit into rigid, short visits in the United States, a more open, flexible schedule of medical appointments would probably be more effective.

- Lewis Culture Category: **Reactive.**

Health Issues and Barriers to Care

- Many Somalis, Ethiopians, Eritreans, and Sudanese are classified as refugees by the United States and are legal residents. As such, they are entitled to a number of health, human service, and economic forms of government assistance for a limited time. Language and transportation can also be significant barriers to care for this group, as can their cultural tendency to delay seeking formal medical treatment until conditions are quite serious and painful.

- Somalia, Ethiopia, and Sudan are among the world's poorest countries. Many immigrants from these nations have experienced significant ethnic conflict, violence, and famine. Many of the East Africans arriving in the United States have undergone profound levels of hardship and human rights abuses, and have personally experienced war injuries, starvation, rape, and torture.

- Many East African refugees had limited access to medical care in their home countries, and often present with multiple physical, dental, and mental health conditions upon arrival in the United States. They tend to view health holistically, in that people should have a balanced life between proper diet, exercise, good family relations, spirituality, their emotions, and other factors.

- East Africans may be unlikely to share with others that they suffer from a mental health condition because of the negative stigma associated with these illnesses, which are usually believed to be caused by negative energy, bad actions, or evil spirits. However, they should be monitored for acculturation stress and post-traumatic conditions such as depression, anxiety, sleeplessness, forgetfulness, flashbacks, nightmares, and the like. Also, the somatization of fear and sadness can result in unexplained physical problems like diarrhea, heart palpitations, general aches, and susceptibility to infections.

- Birth records were not always kept like in the West, and a person's birthday is more likely to be associated with a particular seasonal event than with an exact day and year. Therefore, many East African adults won't know exactly how old they are and won't be able to answer this question accurately on medical forms. At the point of entry to the United States, many immigration officials just estimated the age of each of the new arrivals.

- Many Eastern African newcomers routinely share medications and prescriptions with each other, such as that for tuberculosis.

Also, they often stop taking Western pills once their symptoms stop, even though they might not be through with the full course of medicines. Proper health education programs will need to be created to deal with these topics.

• In general, East African women value breastfeeding, and it may be common for them to nurse their children for two years or more, while also feeding them solid foods. This practice is recommended by the World Health Organization and shouldn't be discouraged by American providers or baby formula marketers. They are also quite adept at nursing their children discreetly in public, and have a rich knowledge of how to overcome nursing difficulties that often stump American women. Encourage the women to maintain their healthy lactation habits and to avoid trying to emulate American women who nurse far less.

• Genital cutting (circumcision) of girls is common in some East African cultures, particularly among those that practice Islam. You will need to become more aware of how to address this topic in a sensitive manner. In the West, this procedure on girls is generally considered to be a form of culturally imposed physical mutilation that can lead to severe infections or even permanent damage to the reproductive organs. However, in cultures where female genital cutting is practiced, this procedure is seen as a valued, highly desirable, and greatly celebrated ritual that usually denotes the passing of a girl into womanhood. Girls who don't participate in this ritual are not likely to be desired as marriage partners and will have little possibility for social and economic power as adult women. Ethnic groups that practice female genital cutting usually feel that this procedure isn't well understood by Westerners and resent the implication that it's a primitive or barbaric practice.

• Clinicians in the United States may be approached by East African refugee mothers who want them to perform circumcisions on their daughters. It is illegal in the United States to perform female genital cutting on patients under 18 years of age, regardless of cultural traditions. Many immigrants know this, and perform this traditional ceremony at home. Because of the highly controversial nature of female genital cutting, you should therefore become thoroughly familiar with the medical and cultural implications of the procedure.

- Many East Africans consider U.S. Americans to be highly wasteful and indulgent, as indicated by the high percentage of people who are overweight. However, in Africa, being heavy is usually a sign of wealth and success, and being underweight is a sign of poverty and poor health.

- East Africans, as a society that values respect and obedience, generally comply fairly well with orders from doctors. However, they tend to be anxious and may resist invasive procedures like surgery.

- East Africans are often stoic in their expression of pain.

Serious Illness and Bereavement

- Bereavement practices vary significantly by East African culture and religion. Many Christians follow similar practices as other Christians in the United States.

- Many East Africans view death as the will of God or spirits. Burial ceremonies are usually meant to appease the spirits so that additional deaths don't occur. They may mourn for a period of several months after a death.

- For Muslim East Africans, burial usually takes place fairly quickly after death. Cremation is usually not practiced. The body is blessed and ritually cleaned in a mosque by an *Imam*, a Muslim religious leader. The body is usually wrapped and then carried, without a coffin, in a funeral procession to the grave. The official mourning period may last between three to seven days.

- East African patients usually don't like to be alone when ill. Large numbers of extended family and friends usually visit ill patients. They may want to spend extended periods of time with them in the hospital, including nights. Visitors often bring meals and other gifts from home. (Hospitals in Africa don't usually provide food for their patients.)

- In general, in times of crisis, East African men are responsible for making important decisions, like which medical procedure should be used with a seriously ill patient or where a funeral should be held. Bad news shouldn't be broken first to women, as they are trained culturally to be more emotionally vulnerable and fragile than men.

- Organ donation and autopsies are usually not allowed by families unless there is a legal or medical necessity.

Traditional Health Practices

- East Africans generally believe that there are multiple causes of poor health. Some illnesses are perceived to have tangible, external causes like a poor diet. However, other conditions are the result of fate, destiny, negative energy, bad spirits, God's will, or the breaking of social taboos.

- Traditional medicines have been used for centuries by East Africans and vary by geography and culture. They are far too numerous to discuss, but be aware that patients will likely be interested in using a variety of herbal, plant, and food remedies if available as a supplement to Western medicine.

- In traditional culture, many East Africans would take care of themselves first at home through common plant and herbal remedies, and not always seek medical attention from physicians. Healers were common in their home communities, but are not readily available in the United States within this immigrant population.

- Muslim East Africans avoid pork in their diet.

- The right hand is considered clean and is used for eating and handshaking; the left hand is considered unclean and is used for cleaning oneself in the toilet and the like. Therefore, be sure to hand items to or touch these patients with your right hand.

- East Africans value balance and harmony among the body, mind, emotions, spirit, family, environment, and universe as the ultimate means to ensure health.

- Many East Africans, such as the Sudanese, practice animism. This traditional form of spirituality recognizes a variety of supernatural beings, including animal and plant spirits. During illness, it isn't uncommon for the Nuer,* for example, to try to determine what evil spirit or bad energy has caused a condition, and then try to rectify it through an offering or an animal sacrifice. The evil eye is also a common belief among this group, whereby a bad person can send negative energy to another and cause misfortune or poor health.

* With a population of about one million, the Nuer are the second largest ethnic group in south Sudan (the Dinka are the largest group) (www.sudan101.com/nur.htm).

EAST ASIAN IMMIGRANTS

Overview

- East Asia is home to some of the world's oldest and most advanced cultures, including China, Japan, and Korea. Large numbers of immigrants from East Asia began arriving in the United States in the 1800s as economic migrants, and they first populated ethnic communities on the West Coast in cities such as San Francisco. Today, East Asian minority communities can be found in all major cities within the U.S., particularly in California, New York, and Hawaii.

- Many East Asians experienced significant levels of discrimination in the United States. For example, in the 1800s racism was rampant against the Chinese laborers who worked to unite the country through railroads. Even into the early 1900s, some businesses regularly placed signs outside stating, "No Chinese need apply." Likewise, during World War II, many Japanese Americans were forcibly sent to live in internment camps in Southern California and elsewhere for fear that they were spies or contributing to the war. Others lost their land and property, or were forced to serve in the military with few rights.

- In general, the Chinese, Japanese, and Koreans who are in the United States have either lived in this country for several generations or are economic migrants.

- East Asians are generally among the least integrated of many minority groups, preferring often to live in ethnic communities with others from their culture.

- Japan and South Korea are among the most highly industrialized and developed countries in the world, and immigrants from these cultures resent being considered primitive or backwards. While China is less industrialized at present, it is now a major trade partner with the United States. China's historic role as a world cultural leader in earlier centuries remains an important source of pride for the Chinese. Likewise, Japan and South Korea have produced some of the world's finest art, literature, philosophy, and religious thought.

• Much diversity exists among East Asians. Chinese, Japanese, and Koreans will be greatly offended if they are assumed to all be the same. In fact, historically, these cultures have often fought each other to retain control of resources and their unique identities. Health programs must be culturally specific for each group.

Language and Religion

• No one language is spoken by all East Asians. Younger Asian Americans, as well as those who were born in the United States, speak English, while Japanese, Korean, or a Chinese dialect may still be spoken by some elders or newer immigrants from those countries. Most East Asians are highly literate.

• Because of the extreme cultural diversity within China, there are many dialects of spoken Chinese, and many of these aren't interchangeable. Mandarin is the most common dialect in all of China, and Cantonese is more common in the south. The written form of the language can generally be understood by most Chinese, regardless of their spoken dialect.

• The religion of East Asians varies by ethnicity and culture. Many today have adopted some form of Christianity. Others still practice the religions that were common in their native countries, such as Buddhism, Zen, and Taoism.

Family and Social Structure

• While East Asians may not have large numbers of children, they nonetheless place great value on the extended family. Each parent and child has a distinct and well-defined role in the family.

Health programs should emphasize the relevance of health issues to family roles rather than on the individual.

- Many East Asians immigrants live in distinct ethnic neighborhoods. They may be somewhat distrustful of outsiders, preferring to rely on others from their own country for assistance. Interventions are best conducted through programs that incorporate health workers from those cultures.

- Gender preferences in children often favor boys in East Asian cultures, although all young children are genuinely adored. They are traditionally taught to be obedient, polite, and subservient when interacting with adults.

- Women are afforded high levels of respect from a familial standpoint, while men are expected to be strong and good providers. Older men are usually recognized as the heads of household, and they serve important roles as spokesperson for the family. Indeed, while the women share their opinions, the men are most often responsible for making final, important decisions, such as those affecting health care. Although many East Asian women work and are highly successful, women are usually still responsible for care of the home, children, and the ill.

Older Adults

- Elders are absolutely revered and valued for their age and wisdom. Children are expected to care for their parents when they age, just like the parents cared for their children when they were young. Multigenerational homes are often preferred, where possible, and East Asians tend to be reluctant to place their elders in nursing homes and other formal care institutions.

- In East Asian cultures, education is held in very high esteem. The majority of elders have completed at least a high school level of education, including some English language training. As a result, seniors are often willing to participate in educational programs.

- Oftentimes, especially with older adults, direct eye contact and a firm handshake can create a sense of confrontation. For this reason, it may be more welcoming to greet elders with a word or phrase in their own languages or with a simple bow. In addition, East Asian elders are normally addressed by their title (*Mr.*, *Mrs.*, *Dr.*, etc.) and not by their first names.

Cultural and Communication Style

- East Asian cultures tend to be fairly reserved and thoughtful when speaking, although their tone of voice may sometimes be animated and loud. In new settings, they can be quite shy.

- East Asians generally place high value on the importance of respect and "saving face." They take great pains not to embarrass or put others in awkward positions. Honor and politeness should be emphasized at all times in interactions between health providers and East Asian patients.

- Direct eye contact, close body spacing, and casual touching aren't very common in East Asian cultures, as a highly defined sense of formality exists in all relations. They tend to be less willing to openly express their opinions or feelings, particularly if they are negative.

- Modesty is extremely important in East Asian culture, particularly among women and the elderly, and you should make every effort to maintain the privacy and dignity of patients.

- Because of the emphasis placed on education and deferential, polite behavior, East Asians may be unlikely to disagree with doctors and other health providers in public. They may nod their heads out of respect, even though they have questions or don't want to comply with a particular medical routine.

- Lewis Culture Category: **Reactive.**

Health Issues and Barriers to Care

- In ethnically distinct neighborhoods, language and culture can be significant barriers to care for East Asian immigrants, particularly those who are older. However, in general, immigrants from East Asia, particularly South Korea and Japan, are well educated, highly literate, and practice many positive lifestyle behaviors. Most have health insurance, particularly if they are American-born minorities.

- Today, Asian Americans have made extreme strides in their standard of living, and generally have an excellent reputation for hard work and educational achievement. Their health status as a group is usually among the very best in the country, often higher than the European American majority, because of genetic factors and positive lifestyle practices. Life expectancies are usually longer, and mortality rates are lower than those for most other cultural groups in the United States. However, with each generation born in the U.S., fewer differences in health status exist. Some health disparities do exist, such as in cervical cancer rates.

- East Asians generally believe that good health is achieved through maintaining balance in all things, such as in interpersonal relationships, diet, exercise, and the emotions.

- Older and less acculturated East Asians tend to be quite modest, so it is generally best to match the gender of the health provider with the gender of the patient, particularly when conducting procedures such as baths or examinations of the reproductive organs. Also, because of modesty, they may delay seeking preventive care such as mammograms, or be too shy to conduct self-care procedures at home, like breast examinations.

- In general, East Asians tend to be stoic in their expression of pain. Also, because of their reserved nature, they may be reluctant to share personal, intimate health information with providers.

- When possible, East Asians generally prefer to avoid invasive procedures such as surgery or the drawing of blood. They value the body being kept intact in its whole, natural state.

- Because of the emphasis that is placed on harmony in traditional East Asian culture, the cause of mental health conditions is often attributed to an imbalance in the emotions. East Asians don't generally distinguish between physical and mental health. Many may be unwilling to seek professional psychological help or to disclose mental illnesses, because of the importance of saving face and maintaining family honor.

Serious Illness and Bereavement

- Bereavement practices vary significantly by culture, ethnicity, and religion among East Asians. If they are Christian, a minister, priest, or other appropriate religious leader should be contacted in cases of serious illness or death. Buddhist patient families may be comforted by a monk. They may also be comforted by lighting incense or practicing other rituals to ensure that the patient's soul proceeds to the proper location in the afterlife.

- Buddhist patients believe that the soul passes through many reincarnations until it is liberated from worldly problems and enters nirvana. As such, death is simply a natural state through which all people pass multiple times. Depending on specific cultural traditions, Buddhists may hold a funeral within several days to a week after death, often with several prayer ceremonies and memorials conducted at home, a funeral parlor, and a temple by a monk or priest prior to burial. Many Buddhists favor cremation over burial.

- Many extended family members and friends will likely visit the ill or deceased patient. To not do so would be considered an insult to the patient's family.

- In general, East Asians tend to be reserved in their expression of grief and sadness in the event of a death, although being visibly distraught and crying loudly isn't uncommon either.

- Asian Americans usually confer great reverence and honor to the departed spirits of ancestors, and regularly honor and remember them through ceremonies and offerings.

- As East Asians believe the body should be kept whole upon death, autopsies and organ donation are generally not allowed.

Traditional Health Practices

- East Asian traditional healing systems are among the oldest and most complex in the world. Many of these techniques have been well documented for thousands of years in standardized texts. In general, they tend to emphasize health from a holistic stand-point: rather than treating a disease symptom, like in the West, they usually emphasize maintaining balance, harmony, and interconnectedness of the body, mind, and spirit.

- East Asian medicine also emphasizes the balancing of what the Chinese refer to as *yin* and *yang* energies. These forces are con-sidered to be polar opposites, but they are both necessary in balance for good health. As many health conditions are perceived to be caused by having too much yin or yang, remedies attempt to rebalance the energy force.

- Moderation is emphasized, and extremes in behaviors, tempera-tures, emotions, and other things are to be avoided.

- East Asian cultures have well-defined usages for many herbal remedies as well. These herbal remedies can be purchased easily from specialty stores in ethnic communities, and shopkeepers are often quite knowledgeable about their historic usage. Note that patients often use these herbal remedies before and while engaging formal Western biomedical care.

- *Chi* is recognized in East Asian culture through various interpretations as the universal life force that permeates all beings. Many traditional East Asian exercises such as tai chi and karate emphasize physical, mental, and emotional states that are conducive to increasing and moving the chi properly through the body for optimal health and productivity.

- Multiple forms of energy healing, like acupuncture and *qi-gong* in China, are used to rebalance the electromagnetic field surrounding living beings. In their health belief system, this rebalancing is necessary to remove blockages of energy that can ultimately cause illnesses and disease.

HISPANICS

Overview

- Latinos now represent the largest minority population in the United States, surpassing even African Americans, according to the 2000 census figures. The Census Bureau predicts that Hispanics will represent close to 25 percent of the U.S. population by 2050. This demographic change is occurring throughout the country, particularly in urban areas and border states. However, rural states have seen some of the greatest increases in Hispanic population growth by town in the U.S.; some communities have increased their percentage of Latinos by 700 percent and even 1,200 percent over the past decade.

- *Latino* usually refers to someone from Latin America, in the Western hemisphere. *Hispanic* usually refers to people who speak Spanish. The U.S. government considers Hispanics to usually be racially white, although of Spanish-speaking origin. Both terms, *Hispanic* and *Latino*, are often used by people from this ethnic group, and the U.S. government recognizes both terms. Many Hispanic immigrants, though, prefer to be identified by their country of origin.

- Most Latinos in the United States have roots in Mexico. Indeed, during the Mexican-American War (1846-1848), Mexico lost almost half of its land to the U.S., so many Mexicans in the Southwest, for example, have been U.S. citizens for four or more generations as a result of this conflict. However, many more have come in recent generations to seek better economic opportunities. The second largest source of Latino immigrants to the U.S. are from other Central and South American nations, such as Guatemala, Nicaragua, El Salvador, Chile, and Argentina. Most have come to the U.S. in more recent decades as either economic migrants or political refugees.

- Two additional significant Hispanic populations in the United States are from Puerto Rico and Cuba, which respectively account for the third and fourth largest Latino groups in the country. Many Puerto Ricans and Cubans immigrated to the U.S. during the 1900s. Puerto Ricans were granted statutory citizenship status from the U.S. in 1917. Many also came to large urban areas like New York in the 1940s. Likewise, Cubans have been coming to the U.S. in significant numbers since the early 1900s to work in agriculture and industry. During the 1960s and 1970s, large numbers of wealthy, educated Cubans fled to the U.S. as refugees from Fidel Castro's communist system, and settled in New York City and southern Florida in immigrant enclaves. More than 100,000 additional Cubans from lower socioeconomic classes, including some criminals, arrived in the U.S. in the 1980s during the well-publicized Mariel Boat Lift.

- It's important for you to recognize the tremendous diversity within Hispanic culture. Cultural practices and Spanish dialects can vary dramatically between and within Hispanic nations because of differences in ethnicity, nationality, and socioeconomic class.

- In addition, significant ethnic diversity also exists among some Hispanic cultures. For instance, among those from the Caribbean, many have intermarried with people of African descent. Others, particularly those from rural areas, may be of indigenous Indian background from their countries, while fair-skinned Hispanics of European descent are common among upper-class and urban populations in South America.

Language and Religion

- Most Hispanics speak Spanish as their primary language, although dialects vary by country and ethnic group. Also, upper-class and lower-class Hispanics may speak somewhat different forms of Spanish. Many second-generation Hispanics in the United States still speak Spanish as their first language, although

English usually becomes the primary language among third- and fourth-generation immigrants. Many Hispanics, though, tend to be proud of their unique heritage and value Spanish for its traditional role in their culture. In fact, Puerto Ricans, for instance, have greatly resented repeated attempts by the U.S. to make English one of the official languages of their island again.

- Most Latinos practice some form of Christianity, with the majority being Catholic. Many Catholic parishes in the United States have now instituted special Spanish-language masses for their new Latino parishioners. Some Latinos may also combine Catholicism with elements of traditional indigenous spirituality from their native culture.

- Many Cubans also practice some form of Christianity, although Fidel Castro encouraged secularism in his communist state. Those Cubans who have been in the United States for longer periods of time may be more likely to practice Catholicism or other forms of Christianity than those more recently arrived.

Family and Social Structure

- Although they often live within nuclear families, Latinos are well known for their extremely strong tradition of extended family. Cousins, for example, are as valued as siblings, while aunts and uncles often serve as second parents. Godparents are also usually very important. Hispanics tend to receive—and expect—tremendous family support. They also have a well-developed understanding of their social roles within the family by age and gender.

- Hispanics usually have a genuine interest in readily participating in activities with the family. The needs of the family are usually placed before those of the individual. Maintaining good relationships with family members is important, and Latinos are generally very affectionate, warm, and loving with each other.

- Although it varies greatly by region, Latino culture places great emphasis on pride and family honor. This is particularly true among males, who are ultimately responsible for maintaining and protecting the family's reputation. However, all family members are expected to behave in appropriate ways to ensure the honor and respectability of the family in public. For this reason, family members may not be willing to report crimes that may carry a negative stigma, such as rape or violence against women.

- Showing respect in human relationships is also critical to Latinos. Thus, make extra efforts to be kind, respectful, and gracious when dealing with Latino clients, to avoid being perceived as having race or class bias when serving these patients.

- Hard work and education are valued in Latino culture. Many Hispanic family members, especially lower-income newcomers, work long hours at multiple jobs to support their families. Financial resources are often shared among family members, and Latino newcomers frequently send large amounts of their salaries back home to relatives in their home country.

- Children are at the center of Hispanic homes and are adored and loved. Traditionally, boys were raised to be strong and protective under social machismo codes. Girls were taught to be more submissive and to play lead roles in maintaining the family and home.

- Increasingly in the United States, Hispanic women are successfully working outside the home. However, most continue the powerful central role of mother, wife, and family caretaker at home as well, although this has caused considerable stress in some cases.

Older Adults

- Age is highly respected in Hispanic culture. Elders are appreciated for their leadership of the family, and they are recognized as sources of wisdom, knowledge, and joy. Seniors are honored and consulted regularly. Aging mothers are particularly influential in health and other decisions affecting the family.

- Elderly Latinos should always be treated with great respect. Address them formally using titles such as *Mr.*, *Mrs.*, and *Sir* unless they request a different greeting form.

- Hispanic seniors may be somewhat reserved and formal upon first contact. It may be helpful to initially "break the ice" with a few Spanish words or phrases at the beginning of a visit. Additionally, it's important to clearly explain the purpose of the appointment, program, presentation, or visit by reviewing information regularly to be sure that clear communication occurs.

- Many Latinos want to take care of their aging parents at home. The family is often multigenerational. Although this is changing now in the United States, the utilization of nursing homes and assisted-living facilities by Hispanics is often seen as a sign that the children don't love their parents and can be considered shameful.

Cultural and Communication Style
- In general, Latinos are an expressive, warm, outgoing, affectionate, and hospitable group. They tend to have closer body spacing and more eye contact with others, and often use more humor, expression, touching, and emotion in their communications than do mainstream white Americans. Try to emulate this warmer style of communication so as to work more effectively with them.

- Respect, honor, and dignity are also important cultural characteristics, as is recognition of social status. Many will show reciprocal acts of kindness for good health care by bringing food or small gifts to providers.

- Privacy and dignity are valued in Hispanic culture. Providers should recognize the importance of maintaining the modesty and confidentiality of patients.

- Face-to-face interactions and family connections are very important in this culture. Health facilities that feature fancy written marketing materials and the latest medical technology will often be less successful than smaller facilities that feature warm, outgoing staff and caring personnel. Many referrals are made by word-of-mouth, particularly in immigrant communities.

- As noted previously, Hispanics greatly value education. Many came to the United States primarily to seek better schooling and greater economic opportunities. They often, therefore, expect the relative with the highest level of education, even a female, to be spokesperson and primary decision maker for the family when health and related issues are at stake.

- Lewis Culture Category: **Multi-Active**.

Health Issues and Barriers to Care

- Money, language, and transportation are usually cited as the major barriers to care for Latinos. A large percentage of newcomers don't have health insurance and lack adequate personal finances to pay out-of-pocket for medical care. Spanish language interpreters may also be difficult to find. Because they often work at two or more jobs if low-income, many Latinos have difficulty using health facilities if they are only open from 9:00 A.M. to 5:00 P.M. Most services aren't located close to where they live, and transportation is usually very limited. Additionally, Hispanic newcomers who don't have the legal documentation to work in the United States often delay or totally avoid seeking medical care, as they fear being reported to immigration authorities and deported.

- Diabetes, occupational injuries, dental care, and acculturation stress are only some of the more common conditions that Latino newcomer patients experience in the U.S. Although this is changing, many Latinos who come to the United States as economic migrants are younger males who are working to help support their families back home. As such, male health concerns and work injuries can be common issues to address, as are maternal and child wellness issues. Increasingly, Hispanic immigrants are bringing their families and parents with them to the U.S., so aging health issues are becoming important as well.

- Fate and destiny are important values in determining patient involvement in disease prevention and treatment activities. Many Hispanics, in particular, feel strongly that God ultimately determines their well-being. As such, many Latinos, particularly those who are less acculturated, may be relatively unwilling to use preventive procedures, such as routine screenings and self-examinations, because of their belief in divine fate.

- Latinos don't always separate physical from mental health, and tend to believe in a more holistic view of well-being. Simultaneously, there is a cultural tendency to view depression, anxiety, and other mental illnesses as embarrassing, dishonorable signs of weakness in the family. As such, Hispanics may not be willing to disclose these conditions to providers and may be reluctant to follow up on referrals to professional counselors and psychologists. They are more likely to rely on their extensive family network for support, care, and comfort.

- Among older or more traditional Latinos, women patients often prefer female physicians for their care. Some Cuban and Puerto Rican women, for instance, delay care out of modesty concerns, especially if the illnesses involve reproductive organs. Likewise, they may be too shy or feel it is inappropriate to conduct self-examinations of the breast for preventive purposes.

• Many Hispanics tend to be quite verbal and expressive when in pain, although the men may be more stoic.

• Hispanic patients usually expect their family members, especially women, to take care of them when they are ill. They may be passive in their rehabilitation and less willing to practice self-care efforts.

• Although this is changing in the United States, the traditional body image valued by Hispanics can vary from that of white European Americans. For instance, Cubans and Puerto Ricans traditionally feel that heavier people are healthier than thin people, who are considered to be weak and sick.

• Health topics such as HIV/AIDS, sexually transmitted diseases, mental conditions, and some birth defects can carry a negative, embarrassing stigma in some traditional Hispanic cultures. Homosexuality may also not be recognized in a family, and can be considered shameful if publicly known.

Serious Illness and Bereavement

• Cultural practices involving serious illness, hospitalization, and bereavement vary among Hispanics by their country and culture of origin. If the Latino patient is Catholic, a priest should be notified if the patient has died or is in very serious condition. Many parishes have priests who speak Spanish and are charged with Latino outreach. The priest will offer special prayers for healing and will perform last rites on a dying patient. Patients' families may also wish to pray themselves, using the rosary or seeking comfort from Jesus, the Virgin Mary, or a saint.

• Most Hispanics who are dying usually expect large numbers of family and friends to visit them. To not do so would be considered an insult. Many extended family members will stay with the dying overnight to provide comfort and care.

- Most Hispanics prefer that dying family members not be informed of having a terminal disease. You will therefore want to consult with the main decision makers for the patient, such as a respected, well-educated, older relative, about the condition first.

- In general, many Hispanics are very expressive when relatives die and may weep loudly or even faint from inconsolable grief as a sign of their loss. Large gatherings of extended family and friends are common at many funerals.

- Cremation is generally not common among this group. In many Latino cultures, the souls of the dead are remembered and honored regularly through religious and community celebrations, such as Day of the Dead parades and offerings in Mexico that run between October 31st and November 2nd.

- Hispanics generally do not support organ donation or autopsies, unless family consensus is obtained and a medical or legal necessity exists.

Traditional Health Practices
- Many individuals, particularly seniors or those of more rural indigenous backgrounds, practice various traditional medicine methods such as herbal healing and energy-cleansing rituals.

- Many Latinos, particularly those who are older, like to combine their traditional health practices with Western medicine. They may be quite adept at making herbal infusions at home with common plants and herbs; many rely on a wide and well-documented variety of plant infusions and aromatic oils for healing, and are willing to share information about these traditional practices when asked respectfully. Many ethnic stores carry these medicinal products over the counter in the herb section.

- Prayer, asking saints to intercede in the healing process, and related spiritual rituals are particularly valued by many Latinos. Fate, destiny, and the divine are perceived to play important roles in the health of patients.

- *Curanderos* are traditional healers in Mexican culture, and are consulted frequently by indigenous tribes and many rural residents back home. In some Latino immigrant communities in the United States, such as small meatpacking towns in rural states, no traditional curanderos are available, and Hispanic newcomers may be reluctant to seek care from local U.S. medical providers.

- Because of the mixing of old- and new-world cultures in the Caribbean, Hispanics from Cuba and Puerto Rico had their own traditional health systems that encouraged harmony among the body, mind, and soul through communication with spirits, the use of medicinal herbs, shamanic rituals, animal sacrifices, magic, and religious practices.

- In Cuba, traditional health practices are closely linked with *Santaria*, which is somewhat related to voodoo and is practiced by a Santero priest. In Puerto Rico, many traditional health practices are a part of *Espiritismo*, a native spiritual tradition from African, indigenous, and Catholic traditions. Traditional Espiritismo healers are called *Espiritistas*. Healers in both religious traditions are sometimes sought in Cuban and Puerto Rican cultural communities when Western medicine is ineffective. Also, these traditional healers can be helpful in addressing conditions considered embarrassing, such as mental illness, which may be viewed as the complex result of negative energy or evil spirits.

INDIANS

Overview

- India, considered by many as a subcontinent of Asia, is the world's 7th largest country. Over one billion residents from a variety of ethnic groups occupy this nation in southern Asia.

- Thousands of Indians have immigrated to the United States since the 1960s for economic reasons, and they reside primarily in large cities throughout states such as California, New York, Illinois, and New Jersey. Most of the Indians who have arrived since the 1960s are highly trained, technical specialists. Immigration laws were eased by the U.S. in recent decades so that shortages in the U.S. labor force in scientific and related jobs could be more easily filled by newcomers like Indians.

- In general, economic migrants to the United States from India are well educated, hard working, and productive citizens. However, as U.S. telemarketing, computer, and service jobs are increasingly being outsourced to India, economic pressures for these workers to migrate to North America, Europe, and other highly industrialized nations might ultimately be reduced.

Language and Religion

- Because India was one of the prime colonies of the British Empire for decades, many Indian immigrants in the United States speak English very well. However, English is only one of India's official languages, with Hindi, Bengali, Sanskrit, and many others also common. Indian immigrants from urban and educated backgrounds are more likely to speak English fluently than those from rural and more impoverished settings.

- Over 80 percent of the population in India practices Hinduism, although Christianity, Islam, and other religions are also present because of the immense diversity within the nation. Hinduism is the world's oldest current religion, having been practiced for more than 4,000 years, and is the third largest religion, after Christianity and Islam.

- Hindus believe in one ultimate god, *Brahman*, which is the principal source of energy that created and maintains all things in the universe. There are also many symbolic deities as well, which affect certain elements of nature and life. Hindus believe in reincarnation. The purpose of life is to live morally in order to ultimately break the cycle of death and rebirth. When this cycle is finally broken, Hindus enter the state of nirvana, where desire is extinguished and the reunion with Brahman is complete.

Family and Social Structures

- Traditional Indian society was based on the well-known caste system of social classes. There were traditionally five castes, ranging from the *Brahmins* (honored and powerful priests) to *Harijans* (the untouchable outcasts). Traditional Indian society had strict behavior codes affecting interaction among the five castes, and individuals remained in the same castes in which they were born. While this caste system has now been legally abolished, it nonetheless permeates many aspects of Indian life. You may find, for instance, that there may be subtle tensions between Indian patients in group settings during cultural interactions, or that interpreter effectiveness might be affected if significant caste differences exist between provider and client. For instance, an interpreter might be uncomfortable asking very sensitive questions of a patient from a much higher caste than himself.

- In general, men are expected to support and protect the family. Traditionally, interactions between the genders were rigidly controlled through social codes, although this is less common among Indians who have been in the United States for a long period of time. Women are expected to play an important role in the family and behind the scenes. Men are more typically responsible for representing the family's opinions and decisions in the public sector.

- The extended family is the basis of Indian society. Members take an active role in caring for each other. Older women, and especially mothers-in-law, can be particularly important in decisions relating to female health. Their traditional influence and involvement may cause some tension among younger and more acculturated Indian families that value independent decision making.

- Men have traditionally been valued over women, and they are expected to maintain the well-being and safety of their mothers, wives, daughters, and sisters.

Older Adults
- Older adults are greatly respected for their age and knowledge in traditional Indian society. In fact, honoring elders is considered a daily duty by Hindus, and seniors are considered a blessing in any gathering.

- Senior women are recognized as being particularly knowledgeable when it comes to family and health matters.

- Aging adults are often taken care of by their children, although families are increasingly seeking institutional assistance in the United States.

- Sons, especially the oldest, are expected to play important lead roles in caring for aging parents. Married sons traditionally lived with their parents, and the elders play active roles in their children's lives. Even today in the U.S., it's not uncommon for Indian parents to move in with their adult children as they age and need assistance.

Cultural and Communication Style

- Indians generally practice a controlled, respectful, and polite communication style. Expressions of pain may likewise be stoic. Public displays of affection and touching are usually not practiced. Emotion is more likely to be shown through the eyes and subtle gestures rather than touch and animated expression.

- From a young age, Indians are raised to be reserved, proper, tolerant, and controlled in their interactions. Shyness and silence tend to be more valued than loud talk and forward behavior. The tone of voice may be quite low.

- Indian Hindu patients will be most comfortable with health providers who are of the same gender.

- Maintaining the modesty and hygiene of Indian Hindus is greatly valued by these patients.

- Direct eye contact between men and women is usually considered forward, unless they are related. Likewise, out of respect, an Indian Hindu man usually won't shake the hand of a woman other than his wife. In traditional mixed groups, health providers should first address the Indian Hindu men before speaking with the women.

- Lewis Culture Category: **Multi-Active/Reactive.**

Health Issues and Barriers to Care

- To the extent that Indians have lived in the United States and have been employed legally for extended periods of time, most have health insurance to cover their needs. Language usually isn't a major barrier, as most speak English.

- Heart disease and sickle-cell anemia are among the more common chronic conditions among Indians who have lived in the United States for a while.

- Indians usually greatly value doctors and other medical providers, and treat them with great respect. To this end, they may be very trusting in the professional opinion of their physician and hesitant to seek alternative opinions or treatments.

- Because of the reserved, proper nature of this culture, Indian patients may be reluctant to share intimate, personal information with unfamiliar health providers until a closer relationship is established. They are more likely to confide in family members and friends about their medical concerns.

- Indian females often prefer to wear their own loose clothes when hospitalized, rather than rely on institutional gowns that they consider to be immodest.

- Foods are classified as either *hot* or *cold* in terms of their energy and effect on the body. Many illnesses are believed to be treated by consuming the opposite food to achieve balance. For instance, one belief is that arthritis, a *cold*, slow disease, is best remedied by eating *hot* foods like yogurt, nuts, and seeds.

- Indians may not disclose mental health conditions to you because of the private nature of their culture. Mental health disorders such as depression are often said to be attributed to spiritual imbalances, or in some cases to evil influences from others. Many believe that excess negative emotions like anger, hate, and fear affect their health. Meditation, yoga, religious prayers, and family support are common ways Indians deal with mental health problems and stress.

- Many diseases and illnesses are believed to be ultimately influenced by *karma*—that negative actions from a previous life may make a person more vulnerable to poor health.

- Good health is believed to be achieved when harmony and equilibrium exist between the various elements that make up the body, mind, emotions, and spirit. Indians believe they have a responsibility to promote their own health and prevent disease through positive lifestyle practices like getting enough sleep, bathing regularly, eating a balanced diet, and praying.

Serious Illness and Bereavement

- Most Indian patients want many members of their extended family to visit them while ill or hospitalized. In cases of serious illness, male visitors such as husbands play a lead role in decision making with the patient, and female relatives may also have input.

- Hospitalized Indian patients tend to be passive and dependent, and expect family members, especially women, to help with their care. The oldest male usually serves as the family spokesperson.

- In times of severe illness, many Indian patients prefer that close family members be notified first of any serious conditions. Some Indian families don't want the patient to be informed about a bad prognosis.

- Because they believe in reincarnation, Hindus recognize the death of the body but not of the soul. They generally accept death with deep understanding and graciousness.

- A Hindu priest may be needed to perform death rites. The oldest son plays an especially important role in death rituals for the father, and the family will want to participate in a final cleansing of the body of the loved one. Health providers should provide privacy for families to perform these last rites.

- Procedures such as organ donation and autopsy are usually not accepted by Hindus, because of their desire to keep the body intact after death for religious regions.

Traditional Health Practices

- Indians have one of the oldest, most advanced, comprehensive, and highly documented traditional health systems in the world. This system, called *Ayurvedic* medicine, emphasizes complete, holistic harmony between the body, mind, and spirit. Within the body, the three *vata*, *pitta*, and *kapha* energy compositions control various physical systems and must be in balance to maintain health.

- Yoga and meditation are two health practices common in the West that have their roots in traditional Indian health.

- Indians have traditionally used an extensive set of Ayurvedic herbs, treatments, and medicines to promote health and prevent disease. Most of these products are meant to provide balance.

- Indian Hindus usually practice nonviolence and don't eat animal products like meat, fish, and eggs.

- As in Muslim cultures, the right hand of Indian Hindus is considered clean and is used for eating and the touching of appropriate or righteous materials. The left hand is unclean and is used for toileting or touching dirty things.

IRANIANS

Overview

- Iran (formerly Persia) is one of the largest countries in the Middle East. In addition to Persians, it has significant ethnic minority populations of Kurdish Iranians, Turkomans, Azerbaijanis, Arabs, and others.

- The people are proud of their long, rich, unique culture that has historically been one of the world's most culturally developed countries.

- Most Iranians began immigrating to the United States in the 1950s, with greater numbers coming since 1979, when the Islamic Revolution occurred. After the revolution, many of the Iranian refugees who arrived in the U.S. were sympathizers or supporters of the Shah of Iran and left because of their unwillingness to live in a fundamentalist religious society.

- Although a diverse group, most Iranians in the United States are highly educated and come from elite professional classes.

Language and Religion

- The primary native language spoken by Iranians is Farsi, or Persian. However, Kurdish, Turkic, Arabic, and English are also prevalent, depending on social class, education, acculturation, and ethnicity. Iran isn't an Arab country in that its people don't speak Arabic.

- Nearly 90 percent of Iranians in Iran are Shia Muslims. The other 10 percent are made up of Sunni Muslims, Christians, Jews, and Zoroastrians.

Family and Social Structures

- Traditional Iranian society is patriarchal. Men are expected to be strong, protective, and good providers, and fathers play important leadership roles in the family. They represent the family to the outside world as the primary spokesperson and decision maker. They can also be excellent caretakers of family members, particularly of their aging parents and children.

- Iranian women are traditionally in charge of the sacred inner world of children and the home. However, even in their home country, women make up a surprising percentage of the doctors, scientists, government workers, and teachers. Today in the United States, Iranian immigrant women are also working successfully outside the home in business, medicine, and other fields.

- The extended family is important in Iranian culture, and children are desired and valued. Iranians usually like to spend extended periods of time with close family members and friends.

- Relationships between family members, friends, and others are highly influenced by complex social rules of interaction and responsibility. Factors such as social class, education, and gender can dictate behavior, for example, in the decisions a family makes regarding the care of its elders or in accepting a certain disease treatment option.

Older Adults

- Older adults are greatly respected for their age and wisdom, and they are frequently consulted for advice and their opinions on important family and social issues.

- Iranian adult children usually want to care for their aging parents at home if possible, although institutionalized care is becoming more popular in the United States. Daughters-in-law are also active in taking care of ill parents, although eldest sons can take lead roles in these issues as well.

- When working with a multigenerational group of Iranians, providers should first greet the oldest Iranians before the younger ones, out of respect.

- Culture and language can still be barriers to care for the elderly.

Cultural and Communication Style

- Iranians generally are an expressive group. Body spacing is often close, and affectionate touching between family and friends is common. Women and men, though, are usually much less comfortable touching each other unless they are married or family members.

- Traditional Iranians are most comfortable with same-sex health providers in order to maintain modesty and privacy, which are important in this culture. In general, Iranians value modesty. Take care to maintain the privacy and dignity of these patients when conducting examinations and other procedures.

- Respect and honor are important cultural traits in Iranian culture. Avoiding shame and embarrassment to the extended family is also crucial. For instance, in a health care setting, be careful about sharing information on mental health diagnoses with the extended family, as these conditions can carry a negative stigma in the culture.

- Because of the value placed on education and social class, most Iranians give great respect to physicians and other health providers. They generally comply fairly well with orders from doctors.

- Lewis Culture Category: **Multi-Active.**

Health Issues and Barriers to Care

- Many Iranians have lived in the United States as refugees for many years, and are a fairly successful immigrant group. Many of them, therefore, have health insurance.

- Iranians are generally quite accepting of Western biomedicine, although they may also have their own cultural understanding of health conditions. For example, handicaps may be understood as being the result of genetic malformations, but also as the result of God's will.

- Health is a subject that is frequently discussed and debated among Iranian families, and advice is freely sought from each other on prevention and treatment options. Home remedies are used frequently before seeking Western medical care. Much like Indian Hindus, good health is often sought through the management and balancing of illnesses with foods.

- Iranian culture recognizes that depression, sadness, and other mental conditions often play out physically in the body. Providers should therefore explore if body aches and pains might not be the result of negative social, personal, or environmental factors.

- Iranians tend to be expressive verbally and physically when in pain. They are usually passive patients, though, and they expect family members to actively care for them.

- As Muslims, Iranians generally avoid pork products. Patients may require special meals that have been prepared to the hygiene standards of their religion. If this option isn't available, families will usually want to bring meals to hospitalized patients from home.

Serious Illness and Bereavement

- Strict Muslims also may not be able to take medicine in gel capsules that have been made out of pork products.

- Iranians, because they are Muslims, view death as the positive beginning of the next phase of existence for the soul. They may grieve more visibly than many Americans do, but tend to be more accepting of death as a natural process.

- Iranians usually do not embalm or cremate.

- Large numbers of family and friends typically visit the dying and the dead. They may want to perform ritual washing of the body upon death, although no religious leader may actually visit.

- The father usually is the main contact and decision maker for the family on death issues. Often, a family won't want a patient to be informed of a terminal illness, for fear that it only creates undo stress in a situation that is ultimately controlled by God's will.

- Iranians generally do not support autopsies or organ donation.

Traditional Health Practices

- Traditional Iranians utilize a variety of herbal infusions and hot-cold food combinations to maintain health and treat simple conditions to manage symptoms, such as mint tea for gastrointestinal upset.

- Iranians usually seek to first treat medical problems at home through self-care and folk remedies. Many ask for the advice and input from other family members and friends before seeking professional help from medical providers.

- In general, there are no traditional healers that play an active role in Iranian immigrant health practices. However, older women often share knowledge with the young on natural remedies.

- Iranians may rely on prayer and spiritual rituals in times of illness, and usually benefit by the active involvement of family in disease prevention and treatment.

JEWS

Overview

- Judaism is one of the world's oldest religions, and was the first major one to recognize one god (monotheism), rather than pantheism (multiple gods). Judaism has been practiced for thousands of years. It eventually gave rise to Christianity 2,000 years ago, and then Islam.

- Jews as an ethnic group originated in the Middle East several thousand years ago, but throughout history have experienced a number of waves of dispersion across Europe, Asia, and Africa due to political upheavals, war, and ethnic cleansing.

- Jewish minorities can be found in many countries throughout the world, including such unlikely nations as China, India, Iraq, and Yemen. Jews have experienced various levels of acculturation in their native countries, with some remaining very devout and isolated, while others have become almost completely assimilated.

- Today in the United States, Jews can be found throughout the entire country, particularly in states such as New York, California, and Florida. Ultraorthodox Jews tend to live in distinct ethnic communities so that they can better practice their religious traditions.

- Jewish immigrants have lived in the United States since the beginning of the country. However, large waves of Jewish refugees came to the U.S. throughout the late 1880s and first half of the 1900s. They fled multiple large-scale religious persecution atrocities and mass human rights abuses, such as the pogroms in Russia and the genocide that occurred during World War II in Nazi Germany, where six million Jews were killed.

- Some hate groups in the Untied States continue to call for Jewish extermination in the U.S., and anti-Semitism is on the rise again in Europe. Most Jews are acutely aware that they have been a persecuted minority throughout history.

Language and Religion

- The native language of Jews in Israel today is modern Hebrew. However, because Jews can be found in many countries throughout the world, they usually speak the native language of that state. Most Jews in the United States speak English as their first language. Many ultraconservative Jews are originally from New York, so they speak English. However, no matter where they are from, most ultraorthodox Jews of European heritage will know some Yiddish, a Germanic language.

- Jews are one of the smallest but most active minority populations in the United States. Jews are extremely diverse among themselves. Those of Western European origin are called *Ashkenazi* Jews, while those of Middle Eastern, Spanish, or non-European origin are called *Sephardic* Jews.

- Jews may be secular or religious. Those who are religious may be reform (not very traditional), conservative, orthodox (very traditional), or ultraorthodox. Among the ultraorthodox, there are various sects such as the Hassidic and the Lubavitchers, which can follow different rabbinical leaders and traditions.

- In Judaism, a person born to a Jewish mother is believed to be a Jew. Most people are therefore born into Judaism rather than convert to it.

- You should be aware of different Jewish calendar issues. Programs shouldn't be operated on the Jewish Sabbath, which begins Friday at sundown and ends Saturday at sundown. Also, don't hold programs during Jewish holidays, such as Passover in the spring, Rosh Hashana (New Year's day in the fall), or Yom Kippur (a day of complete fasting in the fall). Sunday is a working day in Jewish communities. Most Jewish holidays begin at sunset one day and end at sunset one or more days later.

Family and Social Structure

- Most ultraorthodox Jews marry young and have very large families. Reform or more secular Jews have much smaller families.

- Among very conservative Jews, male and female roles are well defined. The men tend to be the heads of household and wage earners, while the women are in charge of the family and home. Many orthodox women are also active volunteers for their community. Among less religious Jews in the United States, a greater level of gender equality exists socially.

- Be respectful of the well-defined gender roles among ultraorthodox Jews. Men should not hug, shake hands, pat the back, or otherwise touch women out of respect. Physical contact between the sexes is usually reserved only for spouses and younger children. Many ultraorthodox men, when passing women in a hall or on the road, typically look down or cover their eyes so as not to infer sexual interest in the women. Ultraorthodox Jewish men may not hide their unwillingness to interact with secular female health professionals.

- Many Hassidic Jewish children study in religious schools. In general, their literacy rates are high. They willingly use technology like computers, cars, and phones.

- Secular and reform Jews usually dress like the non-Jewish majority in the United States. However, ultraorthodox Jews usually wear very modest, dark clothes. Women usually wear long, beautiful dresses or skirts and dark stockings, with their arms fully covered by sleeves, and they use hats or wigs to cover their hair. Ultraorthodox Jewish men wear a *kipa*, or *yarmulke*, which is a skullcap or small covering for the back of the head. This is almost never removed in public. If you work regularly with ultraorthodox Jews, you should take care to dress modestly as well and respect these traditions.

Older Adults

- Jews tend to place a great deal of value on elders, as well as on the generations that came before them. Children are often named after a close family elder who is dead. Family and religious historic traditions are often shared from seniors to the young through stories and during the Jewish holidays.

- Jewish mothers and grandmothers are well recognized for the important role they play in leading the family. They often play very expressive, opinionated, and powerful roles in decision-making issues, especially in topics that affect their children and grandchildren.

- Traditionally, Jewish adults took care of their aging parents at home. Today, many older Jews, especially those who are secular and reform, live in retirement homes or assisted-living facilities that are specifically designed for Jews and cater to their specific dietary and religious needs.

Cultural and Communication Style

- Israelis and Jews in general are extremely warm, passionate, and outgoing people with a sharp sense of humor. Where possible, use this same communication style. Jews also appreciate language that is frank and direct. They are a highly verbal culture that values analytical sparring, so as a health educator, you should be aware that it's often difficult to lecture passively to this type of an audience. Question-and-answer sessions and open discussions are probably more effective.

- Body spacing is usually fairly close in this culture, and physical contact to show affection is common among many Israelis. However, among religious Jews, men and women are generally much more likely to avoid inappropriate contact with each other if they aren't related.

- Where possible, women health providers should work with religious Jewish women clients, and vice versa for men.

- Israelis, like other Middle Eastern populations, place a profound emphasis on respect and hospitality. Health workers will usually need to take the time to discuss other personal issues with this population, before getting down to business with the clients.

- Lewis Culture Category: **Multi-Active.**

Health Issues and Barriers to Care

- Jewish populations in the United States usually don't have significant financial barriers to care. Most American-born reform and secular Jews tend to utilize medical care frequently and early. They usually have insurance, and take an active part in their own care. However, some lower-income Israeli immigrants may not have adequate health insurance if they aren't working legally in the U.S. On the other hand, religious Jews may not feel comfortable utilizing care in the secular or Christian-based hospitals that are common in the U.S.

- Among Jews, health concerns tend to focus on maternal and child topics, obesity, women's health, awareness of genetically based diseases like Tay-Sachs, and prevention of prevalent cancers like those of the breast and reproductive organs.

- From a mental health standpoint, utilization of psychological and counseling services varies by level of acculturation and religious tradition. For example, in this analytical culture where reason and knowledge are valued, reform and secular Jews tend to be quite willing to read about and discuss various mental health conditions that they or their families may have, and generally feel comfortable accessing professional services. In fact, many have pursued careers in this medical health field. However, among very traditional, ultraorthodox Jews, mental health conditions are more likely to have somewhat of a negative stigma attached to them. Their cause and treatment are often attributed to God's will. Large, close circles of friends and family can be very helpful to ultraorthodox Jews in meeting their needs for concern, companionship, prayer, and support.

- Most ultraorthodox Jews usually take an active role in maintaining their own health. They often pool and organize information about the quality of medical providers available to them. There are formal "visiting the sick societies" (*Bikkur Cholim*) that have such information. Bikkur Cholims arrange many facets of community support for patients, including bringing in kosher food, providing companions during medical visits, and communicating with doctors.

- Health providers may experience religious Jews intently probing about the seriousness, necessity, or urgency of a recommended procedure. In some cases, these ultraorthodox patients may feel that the situation warrants consultation with a "high rabbinical" leader. Most ultraorthodox Jews will be very persistent about getting advice from their religious leaders about disease treatment options. Consultation from these rabbinical leaders may result in patients changing a treatment plan or opting for a different medical procedure. If you work with ultraorthodox Jews, don't ridicule this practice; instead, try to work closely with these spiritual advisers who can assert great influence on health decisions.

- Even if no serious health problem exists, consultation by religious Jewish patients with a rabbinical leader often results in his special blessing for good health. The actual outcome of a medical procedure, no matter how it is rated, will be more accepted by the ultraorthodox patient with less speculative hindsight. If the medical situation involves an urgent, life-and-death situation, the patient's family should be informed immediately by health providers of the seriousness of the situation. Sometimes consultation with a high rabbinical leader can be done by telephone rather in person.

- Some patients may bring along a holy book to special procedures. This book is considered by ultraorthodox to be a channel for divine assistance. Many will want to light Sabbath candles as well if hospitalized.

Serious Illness and Bereavement

- Most Jews believe that death ultimately leads to resurrection in a future world.

- Jews usually do not embalm their deceased. Instead, the dead are typically buried within 24 hours of their death, after ritual purification and dressing in a plain linen shroud. The body is usually watched over from the time of death until burial.

- Jews recite the *Kaddish*, a special prayer in honor of the dead. They *sit shiva* for seven days, which means that they curtail most daily activities and mourn out of respect for the dead. During shiva, they often wear black, cover mirrors, and sit on low stools. A special candle is usually lit to honor the dead. The full mourning period lasts one year, at which time a special *yahrzeit* memorial ceremony is held. Religious Jews honor an eleven-month mourning period, and Jews usually celebrate the anniversary of the death of a loved one for many years into the future.

- Many Jews, particularly those of Sephardic background, will be highly expressive and visibly distraught when a loved one dies or is seriously ill. To remain stoic and silent, as is more common in dominant U.S. culture, would imply lack of true feelings for the deceased.

- Autopsies and organ donation are not supported by religious Jews. Less observant Jews may agree to autopsies. Most Jews prefer to be buried with all organs intact.

Traditional Health Practices

- Even nonreligious Jews generally follow some level of kosher dietary laws. These laws emphasize the use of food that is clean and easy to digest, and were first explained by Moses in the Torah, or the book Christians call the Old Testament. Health providers and hospitals, therefore, should be thoroughly familiar with Jewish dietary laws before attempting to discuss nutrition issues or meet their dietary needs. Most Jews won't eat pork or shellfish, and usually don't mix milk and meat products together in the same meal. Israelis, in general, eat far more fresh produce than most U.S. Americans do.

- Religious Jews believe strongly in the power of speech, and words can carry the ability to create destiny through God. With that in mind, they usually don't speak of things that could be considered negative. For instance, they won't usually mention the actual name of a disease like cancer, in that it might give credence to a morbid diagnosis. The families of some very religious Jews or those from some Sephardic backgrounds may prefer that the patient not be told all the details about a serious or terminal disease.

- Most Jews greatly value Western medical care and will access it frequently if financial and geographic barriers don't exist.

- Most Jews usually take an active role in maintaining their own health, and will frequently give advice to others on how to do the same. Many will also question you thoroughly about a particular treatment or medical process, and will expect detailed information.

NATIVE AMERICANS

Overview

- Native Americans are the only indigenous population in the United States, and they are among the most diverse of any minority population in the U.S. The U.S. government recognizes more than 500 separate tribes, or nations, in the country. Most of these tribes have unique and highly distinctive languages, cultures, and practices. Unfortunately, most of the U.S. populace are unfamiliar with their long, rich, and proud history of Native Americans and have had little interaction with them.

- Native Americans can be found throughout the entire United States today. Some European and African American immigrants have family histories that featured intermarriage with Native Americans. Most Native Americans live in urban areas today, as well as on reservations and settlements.

- Native American populations have varying regulations as to how they determine if an individual can receive membership in their tribe. Official enrollment in a Native American tribe can provide a variety of benefits to members, such as health coverage or perhaps a share in casino enterprise profits. Native Americans can usually belong to only one recognized tribe. Many of these groups use *blood quantum* rules, which refer to the amount of *blood*, or Native American heritage a person has, to determine membership (Livesay 2002). Blood quantum rules vary by tribe. For instance, the Cherokee of Oklahoma are the most liberal, while the Ute of Utah require five-eighths minimum blood quantum for enrollment in their tribe. On average, most tribes require a minimum blood quantum of one-fourth. The validity of the blood quantum rule is often debated among Native Americans, and it isn't always recognized as an appropriate way to identify members who may have ethnic or racial heritage from a tribe.

- Like most indigenous populations around the world, Native Americans have, throughout their history, experienced ethnic cleansing, broken treaties, forced displacement, wars, excessive mortality from imported illnesses, legal discrimination, and human rights abuses. Today, although their situation is improving, Native Americans continue to experience some of the highest death and illness rates in the country of any group, and they have the shortest lifespan.

- It is difficult to generalize when working with Native Americans, so health providers should become familiar with the cultural practices of their patients' tribes.

- Try to learn about the unique history of the tribal group or patients you are working with. History texts in the United States are usually written from a white or European American point of view, and many Native Americans understandably have a different viewpoint of key historical events.

Language and Religion

- Most Native Americans today speak English as their primary language, although various indigenous phrases and words are often worked into everyday speech. Native Americans speak the language of their tribe, and over 150 native languages still exist in the United States today. Some elders still know their native language, but many young Native Americans today didn't grow up speaking the language of their ancestors, and must relearn it in special cultural classes in school. Many Native American languages historically had no written form, although the Cherokee, some of the Northeast tribes, and others did.

- There is significant diversity among Native Americans, even within a tribe. Some may be "pure-blooded," while others have family ancestries of intermarriage with whites, Latinos, blacks, or other ethnic groups. From a religious standpoint, many practice some form of Christianity or another religion, others follow Native American spirituality, while others mix both in a unique manner. Native American spirituality isn't considered to be a religion that is "practiced" by indigenous peoples, but rather it's a way of approaching life in a sacred and holistic manner.

Family and Social Structure

- Most Native Americans place great emphasis on family, and genuinely love large numbers of children. In fact, the word in Lakota for children is *sacred beings*. The family, rather than the individual, is the basis of Native American society. The extended family is extremely important and ultimately expands into the tribe. Aunts and uncles often serve as second parents. Depending on the tribe and population, the mother may have multiple fathers of her children, and may not necessarily live with a spouse. Most elders have input and help raise all the children in the community.

- Not all tribes are patriarchal; in fact, a large number are matriarchal. Western providers shouldn't stereotype and assume that women have a low status in their society. Indeed, most Native American cultures place great emphasis on individuality and equality, and the important role that individuals play in contributing to the group.

- Tribal group consensus can be extremely important before undertaking new initiatives or projects. If you wish to establish programs on reservations, for example, you will usually need to meet with multiple parties and ultimately gain tribal council approval before operating programs. Keep in mind that this process can be lengthy.

- Native Americans usually place great value on elders and the practical knowledge they possess. Younger providers should always treat the elders with genuine and sincere respect.

- There tends to be a strong responsibility among Native American culture to bring honor to one's family, tribe, ancestors, and community. It is important not to shame the family through individual actions.

Older Adults

- In traditional Native American society, older adults were revered for their wisdom, knowledge, and advice. They were consulted frequently for advice and input on many important decisions.

- With acculturation, poverty, and the breakdown of traditional Native American society, tension now exists in some families as the influential leadership role of elders has declined. Some seniors openly complain that they feel less useful and valued by younger generations. However, in general, most Native Americans continue to revere their elderly.

- Elderly Native American women can play particularly important roles in decisions that affect the health of the family and the welfare of children and grandchildren. Families were traditionally multigenerational, with adult women and other relatives often caring for aging parents. However, in some Native American communities, assisted-living facilities and group homes have now been established to care for the elderly. Urban Native American seniors can frequently live particularly lonely lives, with few relatives and friends available close by for support.

Cultural and Communication Style

- From a communication standpoint, Native American culture tends to be reserved, thoughtful, and subtle in the direct expression of feelings and thoughts. The tone of voice is usually calm, quiet, and polite. Conversations may have long pauses to allow time for silent reflection.

- Saving face and avoiding conflict can be important in many of the tribal cultures. Ask open-ended questions, and allow Native patients adequate time to respond without interruption. Rather than using direct statements, Native American speech often uses metaphors, stories, and examples to make a point.

- Body spacing tends to be distant and direct eye contact is often avoided as a sign of respect and honor.

- Like many nonWestern cultures, Native Americans generally place less emphasis on time than mainstream U.S. Americans do. You shouldn't expect that all appointments will be kept or that your patients will always call to cancel or reschedule. Flexible, open scheduling is probably better with this population if possible.

- Most Native American cultures value face-to-face informal education and interaction over written, formal information. Storytelling, particularly with younger Native American audiences, can be a valuable health education tool.

- Lewis Culture Category: **Reactive.**

Health Issues and Barriers to Care

- Many Native Americans have difficulty accessing medical care in the United States for a variety of reasons. Because many are impoverished, they have limited financial means to purchase services, unless they are provided free or at low-cost by organizations operated by the Indian Health Services (see Part 5 for contact information) or individual tribes. Transportation and geographic barriers are also significant, particularly if the Native Americans live on large, sparsely populated reservations with few medical providers. Culturally, many Native Americans value their traditional healing practices and often don't feel comfortable seeking care from hospitals or white providers.

- Native Americans suffer disproportionately from many diseases and conditions, particularly diabetes, obesity, alcoholism, accidents, suicide, and murder. Their morbidity and mortality rates for many such conditions and illnesses are among the worst in the country.

- You will need to allow adequate time to establish a close, trusting relationship with Native American patients. Before conducting health visits, take time to get to know the clients as people, rather than just as patients. When working on a reservation or with a clearly defined group of Native Americans, it is also helpful to be invited into the group by one or more of them; however, it tends to be somewhat difficult to "break into" this culture because of the importance of trust and personal relationships.

- Many Native Americans are skeptical and suspicious of putting their signatures on written forms because of a history of broken treaties and the like with the U.S. government. As such, when asking for written consent and signatures on medical papers, check with Native American patients to see if they would like family members to assist in reviewing the forms or making health care decisions.

- In many Native American communities, the modern diet consists largely of starchy foods, refined carbohydrates, and high-fat products. Consumption of fresh produce and healthier, more traditional foods isn't always common due to a variety of factors, such as limited incomes, availability, and acculturation.

- Mental health conditions among Native Americans may be expressed in vague physical symptoms such as aches, pains, and lethargy. They may believe that mental illnesses are caused by patient disharmony with the environment, the spiritual world, or personal relationships. In some Native American cultures, mental imbalances may be considered the result of violations of cultural prohibitions, negative energy, or evil spirits.

- Most Native Americans face pain quietly and very stoically. Spiritual practices and traditional religious rituals can often bring comfort.

- Never remove any amulets, medicine bags, feathers, or other such traditional items from Native American patients unless absolutely necessary. Get permission first from the patients or their families to do so, and the items should be handled with great respect and care.

- The utilization of preventive health measures like screenings varies by ethnicity, education, acculturation level, gender, and the like. While some Native Americans may be quite willing to access preventive services, those who are more traditional don't recognize disease until it actually manifests itself.

- Native Americans recognize a variety of treatments for diseases. Some conditions, such as diabetes, are seen as illnesses that were introduced to indigenous cultures by foreigners. To this end, Western medical care is often considered to be most appropriate for treatment. However, many Native Americans feel that other conditions, such as depression or anxiety, may be best treated through traditional medicinal, spiritual, and ritual purification practices.

- Alcoholism rates are often rampant among many Native American populations. While Western providers may view this as an addictive disease that is the result of genetic susceptibility, some Native Americans consider it to be a severe reaction to the loss of culture, identity, and indigenous soul that occurred because of domination by white society.

Serious Illness and Bereavement

- The bereavement practices of Native Americans are as diverse as the tribes and religions from which they come. It is therefore extremely hard to generalize for this group. Make an effort to learn as much as you can about the Native American patient while he or she is still well enough to communicate, so as to avoid any cultural misunderstandings during severe illness or upon death.

- Some Native American families prefer that patients not be told of serious illness, and these loved ones take an active role in decision making for the sick and dying. In other tribes, greater autonomy and independence from the group is more often the case, and the individual patient is expected to make all appropriate health care decisions.

- In general, many extended family members and friends visit the ill or deceased patient. If the patient or family is fairly traditional, a variety of ritual healing and purification ceremonies may be conducted with the patient. Many of these ceremonies will be communally performed. Often, powerful herbs such as sage are burned as a method of ceremonial purification and harmonizing.

- Open expressions of grief and sadness may be somewhat reserved in this population. Indeed, mourning isn't usually displayed in the presence of the patient.

- Family meetings at the end of life are helpful to determine the wishes and beliefs of the patient regarding funeral arrangements.

- The spirits of the dead in most Native cultures are honored regularly for generations. Most consider death to be merely the beginning of another journey into the next world. The patient's loved ones often have particular dietary, spiritual, and behavioral practices which they must follow for set periods of time while grieving for the dead. Even if the patient is Christian, many will interweave elements of Native American spirituality into the funeral, such as placing sacred herbs or prayer ribbons near the grave.

- Most traditional Native Americans do not support autopsies or organ donations.

Traditional Health Practices

- Indigenous populations around the world are known for their strong sense of connection to the earth and the universe, and their corresponding respect for all living and nonliving things. They tend to understand in a very holistic manner the place of humans in the broader scheme of life. People are traditionally viewed as not being any more or less important than any other living thing, and thus should be responsible caretakers of the self, the family, the tribe, and the earth. Before *sustainable development* was ever coined as a term in Western culture, Native Americans were emphasizing the importance of not doing anything harmful to the environment that could affect future generations.

- Native Americans have a well-developed traditional health system that is very holistic, combining physical, mental, emotional, and spiritual well-being. Physical problems are understood as usually being caused by emotional, mental, or spiritual imbalances. Hence, harmony and a sense of balance in all things, including mind, body, spirit, and the environment, are important for wellness. As such, Native American health beliefs tend to be more circular and indirect in comparison to the more linear "cause-and-effect" view of Western medicine. Native American healing cannot be separated from spirituality. This spirituality is different from religion, and emphasizes the interconnectedness, sacredness, and balance of all things.

- Many Native Americans combine Western medicine with traditional medicine practices, like using herbal remedies, participating in a healing ceremony with a medicine man, performing ritual purification and sweating ceremonies, and other practices. They recognize that Western medicine may be powerful for treating disease symptoms in the body, but generally feel that Native American healing is ultimately best for the soul. Try to learn as much as you can from the local healers who work with the Native American clients, but keep in mind that many of these healers are unwilling to readily share this information because of its sacred nature and a lack of trust of outsiders.

PACIFIC ISLANDERS

Overview

- The nations and cultures that live on the islands of the vast expanses of the Pacific Ocean are among the most diverse in the world. In general, these island people are broken into three categories: Polynesian, Micronesian, and Melanesian. They come from a broad array of countries and locations, including sites as diverse as Hawaii, Tahiti, Samoa, Tonga, Fiji, and New Zealand.

- Although some Pacific islands remain uninhabited, most have been colonized or occupied by European or American powers over the past few centuries. As such, their history in many ways mirrors that of Native Americans and other indigenous populations around the world. Many of these native Pacific Islanders died in previous centuries due to conflict, exploitation, and the introduction of foreign diseases. Many have also intermarried with people of European and East Asian descent.

- Today, nearly 12 million individuals reside throughout the Pacific islands. The vast majority of the roughly 500,000 Pacific Islanders living in the United States, though, are Polynesians from Hawaii, Samoa, and Tonga. Immigrants from Guam and Fiji can also be found in the U.S. Nearly half of the Hawaiians and other Pacific Islanders in the U.S. live in California.

Language and Religion

- Pacific Islanders are among the most linguistically diverse people in the world. Most of these who live in the United States speak English. Many are no longer familiar with the native language of their indigenous culture, and some will mix a few native words with English in a pidgin dialect.

- Religion varies by ethnic group. Many Pacific Islanders in the United States today practice some form of Christianity such as

Catholicism. Others, particularly if they have intermarried with East Asians, may practice Buddhism. Still others may follow their own native spiritual traditions or practice a blend of religions. Those who follow traditional native spirituality recognize a variety of spirits and supernatural powers as playing important roles in the lives of people.

Family and Social Structure

- Pacific Islanders usually value large families, and the extended network of cousins, aunts, uncles, and grandparents is central to their culture. All take an active part in raising the children.

- Like most native peoples, Pacific Islanders have a strong connection between self, the family, the land, the universe, and divinity. Long after they immigrate, they continue to maintain a strong relationship with their native land.

- Pacific Islanders usually have well-defined roles for family members based on age and gender. For instance, children are adored and desired, but typically are expected to know that their role in the culture is subservient to their elders.

- In some Pacific Island cultures, such as Samoa, traditional tribal leaders like the *matai* continue to play important decision-making and social leadership roles in immigrant communities. They are sometimes consulted when health decisions must be made.

Older Adults

- Although children are absolutely adored, they are thoroughly expected to understand their role in society. As such, they have significant obligations to honor, respect, and take care of their elders at all times.

- Many extended family members, especially older adults, live together as multigenerational households. The interdependence of family members is recognized, encouraged, and honored.

- Older adults are held in high esteem and are highly respected. They are always greeted formally with titles of *Mr.* or *Mrs.* They may also be greeted with the title of *Aunt* or *Uncle*, even when no blood relationship exists.

Cultural and Communication Style

- Pacific Islanders usually value harmony and politeness in their interactions with each other.

- Many Pacific island cultures are deferential to medical providers. Out of respect, they may avoid direct questions or confrontational situations. Saving face and handling themselves courteously is important.

- Because of their quieter and more reserved style of communication, Pacific Islanders are often stoic in their expression of pain. Also, discomfort is viewed to be the result of God's will.

- Direct eye contact is sometimes avoided out of respect, particularly if someone is speaking in front of a group for the first time.

- Lewis Culture Category: **Reactive.**

Health Issues and Barriers to Care

- Culture may be the most significant barrier to care for many Pacific Islanders in the United States, particularly as many are U.S. residents and have health insurance.

- Many Pacific Islanders suffer from high levels of obesity, diabetes, and heart disease. Others experience significant rates of female cancers due, in part, to late diagnoses of the diseases.

- Acculturation and the loss of traditional native identities have also contributed to depression, alcoholism, and substance abuse in some communities. The somatization of general aches and pains may be the result of unspoken mental health conditions like depression and anxiety. Patients with mental conditions usually need and want additional attention and support from their large, extended families.

- Pacific Islanders believe they are in good health when their physical body is in harmony and balance with the family, the environment, and the spirit world. Because of their holistic view of health, treatment plans should also promote comprehensive strategies that address the mind, emotions, and spirit.

- Some Pacific Islanders may be too reserved to feel comfortable conducting self-examinations at home of private body parts, such as breasts, for preventive reasons. As such, they may miss early detection of some diseases and can ultimately present with advanced illnesses.

- Similarly, some Pacific Islanders delay seeking care from doctors and clinics due to cultural, language, and financial barriers to care, particularly for preventive issues, and thus ultimately present with more advanced medical conditions.

- Because of their shy, respectful nature when around figures of authority, many Pacific Islanders may indicate that they agree with a physician's opinion, even though they do not. They may likewise be too intimated by health providers to ask questions.

- Some Pacific Islander groups view larger bodies as being healthy and beautiful. They are likewise sometimes encouraged to eat large portions of food to achieve this look.

- Pacific Islanders tend to be fairly modest and generally feel uncomfortable in typical hospital gowns. They may prefer to wear their own loose clothes for privacy purposes.

Serious Illness and Bereavement

- Like many indigenous cultures, Pacific Islanders usually view death as a natural consequence of life. They tend to be more reserved in their expression of sadness when a loved one dies.

- Pacific Islanders usually honor and remember the spirits of ancestors and the deceased. Some believe their own souls will be united with those of their deceased ancestors in the future. They usually appreciate private time to be with the dying, and may want to participate in special death rituals to recognize the soul of their dead loved ones.

- Family members usually prefer to be actively involved in the care of sick relatives. Many may come from far distances to visit the ill in hospitals or to care for them at home.

- Pacific Islander families often prefer that all members participate in health care and related important decisions through consensus in an egalitarian manner.

- In general, Pacific Islanders usually are reluctant to support organ donations or autopsies.

Traditional Health Practices

- Many of these cultures had their own traditional healers who combined herbs, prayer, specialized massage, and shamanism to rebalance patients' health. Today, these traditional healers are still available in some locations and can be helpful to clients while they also use Western medicine.

• As some Pacific Islanders are strongly Christian, they may participate in a variety of prayer rituals and religious services for the ill.

RUSSIANS AND EASTERN EUROPEANS

Overview

- A number of immigrants from Russia and other republics that formerly comprised the Soviet Union live in the United States. Many of them are economic migrants. While they may once all have been part of the former U.S.S.R., they are nonetheless fairly diverse in a number of areas. Don't assume that they are all "Russian," as a number of them are actually from Ukraine, Latvia, Belorussia, or other republics.

- Five major waves of Russian immigration have occurred in the United States since the early 1900s. From 1900 to 1914, many Eastern Orthodox Christian Russians fled to the U.S. to seek religious freedom and greater economic opportunities. Many more thousands came to the U.S. between 1918 and 1940 from Russia's upper class, as a result of the Bolshevik revolution. In the middle of the 1900s, about 20,000 Russian war prisoners arrived from Germany. Nearly 200,000 Russian Jews sought refuge in the U.S. as political and religious dissidents in the 1970s and 1980s. With the beginning of the dissolution of the Soviet Union in 1989, thousands of additional immigrants started coming to the U.S.

Language and Religion

- Most of the immigrants from the former Soviet Union speak Russian, a Slavic language, although they may also know the specific languages of the republics where they used to live, like Ukrainian. Russian is written using the Cyrillic alphabet, which is different than the Latin alphabet used for English.

- Religion varies by ethnic group. Some Russians are quite secular, having been raised in the former Soviet Union where organized religion was discouraged. Others practice some form of Christianity like Eastern Orthodox, while others are Muslim.

Family and Social Structure

- Although most Russians live in nuclear families in the United States, they still continue to have very strong extended family ties. Health services that target the entire family can be especially valuable. Russians may have fewer children in comparison to other immigrant groups from non-Western nations.

- In general, immigrants from Eastern Europe place great value on education, art, music, and fine culture. Although some may be working today in the United States in blue-collar jobs, many were professionals back in their home countries. They therefore are fairly literate, although perhaps not in English, and resent being treated as backward or uneducated immigrants.

Older Adults

- In the Russian culture, there is a sense of naturalism about the end of life. At a young age, the idea is established that living a naturally healthy life will help a person to achieve wellness. For this reason, if a person is diagnosed with a terminal illness, it is often the decision of the entire family whether to tell the dying person of their illness, helping to keep the end-of-life experience as peaceful as possible.

- Older adults are held in high esteem and are greatly respected. Russians almost always greet elders formally with titles of *Mr.* or *Mrs.*, and they may also use the title of *Aunt* or *Uncle* even when no blood relationship exists.

Cultural and Communication Style

- Russians usually are highly verbal, analytical, and fairly direct in their communications with other people. Their tone of voice can be loud and expressive at times.

- Most Russians are extremely literate, well educated, and very knowledgeable about culture, economics, world history, and current affairs. Many enjoy intellectual conversations, and may expect you to know about and discuss world affairs with them, in addition to any health issues that need to be reviewed.

- Eye contact among Russians tends to be direct. Greetings among friends and family are usually loving and expressive. Touch is used frequently, too, as a sign of affection. Body spacing can be more formal and distant when interacting with health providers, but quite close when interacting with loved ones.

- Lewis Culture Category: **Multi-Active.**

Health Issues and Barriers to Care

- Cost, language, and transportation are the most significant barriers to care for immigrants from the former Soviet Union. Many work at jobs that don't provide health insurance, and few medical organizations have Russian interpreters. Others find it difficult to attend health clinics that are only open Monday through Friday during the daytime, since many new immigrants are working several jobs and have limited free time for off-site services.

- For cultural reasons, many won't seek formal medical care, except in more complicated cases. Instead, they typically use some form of self-treatment before ultimately contacting a physician for care if they continue to be ill. Russians usually take an active role in maintaining their own health.

- Mothers are particularly involved in caring for their children's illnesses with alternative therapies. Many Russian immigrant women, particularly those who studied education in universities back home, have had significant training in primary health skills as part of their curriculum.

- Smoking and alcohol consumption rates are fairly high among Eastern European immigrants in general, and are an integral part of their culture. Many Russians, particularly men, are able to consume large amounts of alcohol gracefully, without obviously appearing to be intoxicated.

- The former Soviet Union had a comprehensive, free national health care system for all residents, and elements of this system continue today in the independent republics. Many of the Eastern European newcomers to the United States have little understanding of U.S. concepts of private party insurance, fee-for-service care, and other elements. Many will need assistance navigating the health care system in their new community, and will often seek Russian-speaking physicians if they are available.

- Mental illnesses generally carried a strong negative stigma in the former Soviet Union, where these conditions were often treated by forced institutionalization under KGB supervision. They were often not even discussed among families with members suffering from various conditions. Many Eastern European immigrants are therefore still reluctant to openly admit to feelings of depression, anxiety, acculturation stress, and other mental health challenges that are very normal among newcomer populations. Be aware that these conditions may exist in these patients, and that you may need to approach this subject tactfully and with full confidentiality.

- Russians tend to be very stoic in their expression of pain. You may need to offer pain medication, even if patients don't request it.

Serious Illness and Bereavement

- For those Russian immigrants who are Eastern Orthodox Christians, most believe that death is a necessary consequence of life, and that they will achieve eternal life in heaven if they have lived a good and proper life.

- Eastern Orthodox Christian religious leaders typically hold a special vigil over the deceased, called *panikhida*. This special contemplative time includes prayers, hymns (*tropar*), chants, frequent repetition of the name of the deceased, and readings from the Christian gospel.

- Many family members and friends will likely visit the seriously ill and deceased. They may join in special prayers for the dead, where they ask for mercy on the soul of the deceased patient.

- Burial of the body is far more common than cremation. However, cremation is not prohibited. Many Russian immigrants choose to be cremated in the United States, so that their ashes can be transported back home to Russia.

- Most Russians do not support autopsies or organ donations.

Traditional Health Practices

- Eastern Europeans from the former Soviet Union have a long history of using traditional herbal remedies for care, which they often did in conjunction with their standard Western medical treatments. Many elderly Russians continue to have a strong interest in utilizing homeopathic remedies, herbal teas, and alcoholic tinctures to treat disease and promote health. While U.S. Americans may consider this alternative medicine, remember that herbal medicine is a traditional form of care used by generations of Eastern Europeans.

- Russians may also bring medical kits with them from home that contain a variety of drugs to treat general ailments such as headaches, indigestion, bacterial infections, and the like. Most of these medicines are available over the counter in Russia, but they would require prescriptions in the United States. Be sure to respectfully ask and try to understand the types of self-treatment your Russian clients may be using.

- The main goal of health care in the former Soviet Union was usually finding the root causes of a particular disease or condition. Many Eastern European immigrants to the United States feel that U.S. doctors, on the other hand, place too much emphasis on treating the disease, rather than trying to understand its causes from a more holistic standpoint. Most Russian patients like to have active discussions with their providers about what caused their ailments.

SOUTHEAST ASIAN REFUGEES

Overview

• Southeast Asia comprises a diverse group of nations such as Thailand, Vietnam, Laos, Cambodia, the Philippines, and Indonesia. These countries are very heterogeneous, and have many distinct cultural minorities within them such as the *Hmong* and *Tai Dam* who inhabit the Indochina region.

• Many Southeast Asians arrived originally in the United States during the 1970s and 1980s as refugees from the war in Indochina. Most of these immigrants from Vietnam, Cambodia, or Laos were officially declared refugees and thus were entitled to certain resettlement benefits from the U.S.

• Most of the Southeast Asian refugees who came to the United States in the 1970s were well-educated professionals, especially those from Vietnam. Those who came in the 1980s were given the derogatory name of *boat people*, because they often fled Southeast Asia at great risk on the open sea in rafts, were less educated, and poorer than those who came a decade earlier. Many of them came from countries such as Laos and Cambodia.

• Because of their official refugee status and the political upheaval they experienced during the Vietnam War, many U.S. communities welcomed large numbers of Southeast Asian refugees into their cities and towns in previous decades, and provided them with organized health and resettlement services.

Language and Religion

• No one language is spoken by all Southeast Asians. Younger Southeast Asians, as well as those who have been in the United States for several generations, usually speak English. However, many still know the language of their original homeland, or phrases from it. This could be Vietnamese from Vietnam, Khmer from Cambodia, and others. At the same time, some elderly

Southeast Asian refugees, such as those from Vietnam and Laos, may know French or other European languages from the days of the colonial powers that formerly influenced their countries.

• Some Southeast Asian refugee groups, particularly if they are older, may have low literacy rates in their own language as well as in English. For instance, the Hmong refugees, who were rural hillside dwellers in Southeast Asia, didn't have a written language until the 1950s, and not all had opportunities to attend school.

• The religion of Southeast Asians varies by ethnicity and culture. Many today have adopted some form of Christianity and may be Catholic. Others still practice the religions that were common in their native countries, such as Buddhism. Others like the Hmong may be animists.

Family and Social Structure

• Many Southeast Asian refugees, particularly in larger communities, live in distinct ethnic neighborhoods. They tend to rely on each other and their extended families for support. They can be somewhat distrustful of outsiders and fairly private in their matters.

• Southeast Asian families can be quite large, with members having clearly defined roles according to their age and gender. The extended family is extremely important.

• Young children are genuinely adored, valued, and loved. Women are afforded high levels of respect from a familial standpoint. Many Southeast Asian cultures place great emphasis on the power of women, who often run small businesses in addition to being the primary caretakers of the home and children. Adult men and the oldest sons play important decision-making roles in society, and women may be more deferential to men on these matters.

- Also refer to the section "East Asian Immigrants," as most family and social structure issues are quite similar.

Older Adults

- Elders are highly revered, honored, and valued for their age and wisdom.

- Many Southeast Asians prefer to take care of their elders at home, rather than use formal assistance such as nursing homes. A cultural expectation exists that children will care for their aging parents, just as the adults once cared for their own children. This isn't seen as a burden, but as an obligation and courtesy.

- Older adults usually prefer to be addressed by title (for example, *Mr.* or *Mrs.*) plus their family name, rather than by their first name, out of deference.

Cultural and Communication Style

- Most Southeast Asians tend to be more reserved and quieter than European Americans. They may not mention any dissatisfaction, but they may not return to a health facility if they are upset with the care they received.

- Southeast Asians usually avoid prolonged, direct eye contact and close body spacing as a sign of respect to others. A well-defined sense of formality exists in all relations. A slight bow may be a more appropriate form of initial interaction between provider and patient.

- Southeast Asians are less likely to be confrontational with others, and generally don't like to argue in public. Hence, patients may be unwilling to disagree with you or ask questions. A nod may imply that the patient heard what you said, but it doesn't necessarily mean that he or she intends to comply with it.

- Because of the nature of large extended families in Southeast Asian cultures, private patient information may not always remain confidential, particularly if younger members are interpreting for older adults.

- Modesty is extremely important in Southeast Asian culture, particularly among women and the elderly, so you should make every effort to maintain the privacy and dignity of patients.

- Lewis Culture Category: **Reactive.**

Health Issues and Barriers to Care

- In refugee neighborhoods, language and culture can present significant barriers to care for Southeast Asians. Health programs should always be appropriate for the specific target population because of the differences in language and culture. For older and less acculturated Southeast Asians, the use of interpreters is very important.

- Because of their official refugee status, most Southeast Asian immigrants from Indochina had financial access to medical care when they arrived in the United States. Today, many are integrated into U.S. society and have health insurance through their jobs.

- Refer to the section "Health Issues and Barriers to Care" for East Asian Immigrants, as these are quite similar for Southeast Asian refugees.

Serious Illness and Bereavement

- Bereavement practices vary significantly by culture, ethnicity, and religion among Southeast Asians. A Christian minister, Catholic priest, Buddhist monk, or animist shaman may be helpful to the patient in times of serious illness or death.

- If the patient is Buddhist or animist, the family will place great emphasis on ensuring that the soul of the departed finds its proper way into the afterlife. They may light incense or perform other rituals.

- Large numbers of extended family and friends will likely visit the ill or deceased patient. Some may want to sleep in the hospital for long periods with the sick patient, or may bring meals and practical gifts from home.

- In general, Southeast Asians are less openly expressive about their grief and sadness in the event of a death, although some may be visibly distraught.

- Southeast Asians usually confer great reverence and honor to the departed spirits of ancestors, and regularly honor and remember them through ceremonies and offerings.

- In general, Southeast Asian families prefer to protect very ill patients from knowing the seriousness of their conditions. Families should be involved in any consent and information procedures whenever possible before involving the patient.

- In general, Southeast Asians do not support autopsies or organ donations.

Traditional Health Practices
- Southeast Asian traditional healing systems can be quite similar to those practiced by many East Asians, especially the Chinese. In general, they tend to view health from a holistic standpoint, and emphasize the interconnectedness of the body, mind, and spirit. Balance and harmony in emotions, lifestyle behaviors, dietary practices, work, and other matters are important to ensure good health.

- In traditional Southeast Asian cultures, some illnesses are believed to be caused by imbalances in the human energy field or soul, and may even be affected by spirits from previous lives. Special amulets may be worn at times to ward off evil spirits and influences, and to protect their well-being.

- Where imbalances in energy occur in the body, Southeast Asians may practice traditional methods of relieving this blocked negative energy. For example, if a certain area in the body is causing illness, they may free this discomfort by pinching or rubbing coins over the affected area, or placing heated cups on the skin to create suction. These ancient practices often leave tell-tale bruises or marks on the skin that can be misinterpreted by officials as child abuse or domestic violence.

- Like their East Asian counterparts, Southeast Asian refugees often use traditional herbal remedies as alternative and complementary forms of medicine to Western care. Chinese herbs are particularly valued.

PART 5

Resources

NATIONAL RESOURCES ON MINORITY, IMMIGRANT, AND REFUGEE HEALTH

Asian & Pacific Islander American Health Forum
450 Sutter Street, Suite 600
San Francisco, CA 94108
Telephone: 415-954-9988
Fax: 415-954-9999
E-mail: healthinfo@apiahf.org
Website: www.apiahf.org

Centers for Disease Control and Prevention
1600 Clifton Road
Atlanta, GA 30333
Telephone: 800-311-3435
Website: www.cdc.gov

Closing the Health Gap
P.O. Box 37337
Washington, D.C. 20013-7337
Telephone: 800-444-6472
E-mail: HealthGap@omhrc.gov
Website: www.healthgap.omhrc.gov

DiversityRx

E-mail: rcchc@aol.com
Website: www.diversityrx.org/HTML/DIVRX.htm

Indian Health Services

The Reyes Building
801 Thompson Avenue, Suite 400
Rockville, MD 20852-1627
Website: www.ihs.gov

International Organization for Migration (IOM)

17, Route des Morillons
CH-1211 Geneva 19 - Switzerland
E-mail: info@iom.int
Switzerland
Telephone: +41-22-717-9111
Fax: +41-22-798-6150
E-mail: hq@iom.int
Website: www.iom.int

The National Alliance for Hispanic Health

1501 Sixteenth Street, NW
Washington, DC 20036
Telephone: 202-387-5000
E-mail: alliance@hispanichealth.org
Website: www.hispanichealth.org

National Institutes of Health
National Center on Minority Health and Health Disparities

6707 Democracy Blvd., Suite 800
MSC-5465
Bethesda, MD 20892-5465
Telephone: 301-402-1366
Fax: 301-480-4049
Website: www.ncmhd.nih.gov

Office of Minority Health

P.O. Box 37337

Washington, DC 20013-7337

Telephone: 800-444-6472

Fax: 301-251-2160

Website: www.omhrc.gov/omhhome.htm

Refugee Health and Immigrant Health

E-mail: Charles_Kemp@baylor.edu

Website: www3.baylor.edu/~Charles_Kemp/refugees.htm

United Nations High Commissioner for Refugees

Case Postale 2500

CH-1211 Genève 2 Dépôt

Switzerland

Telephone: +41-22-739-8111

www.unhcr.ch/cgi-bin/texis/vtx/home

United States Department of Health and Human Services

Office for Civil Rights

200 Independence Avenue, SW

Room 509F, HHH Building

Washington, DC 20201

Telephone: 800-368-1019

TDD: 800-537-7697

E-mail: ocrmail@hhs.gov

Website: www.hhs.gov/ocr/mission.html; www.medicare.gov

NATIONAL RESOURCES ON MINORITY AGING ISSUES

Administration on Aging
Washington, DC 20201
Telephone: 202-619-0724
E-mail: AoAInfo@aoa.hhs.gov
Website: www.aoa.gov

National Asian Pacific Center on Aging (NAPCA)
1511 Third Avenue
Suite 914
Seattle, WA 98101
Telephone: 206-624-1221
Fax: 206-624-1023
Website: www.napca.org

National Association for Hispanic Elderly
234 East Colorado Blvd., Suite 300
Pasadena, CA 91101
Telephone: 626-564-1988
Fax: 626-564-2659
E-mail: support@anppm.org
Website: http://anppm.org

The National Caucus and Center on Black Aged, Inc.
1220 L Street, NW, Suite 800
Washington, DC 20005
Telephone: 202-637-8400
E-mail: info@ncba-aged.org
Website: www.ncba-aged.org/index.html

National Hispanic Council on Aging

341 Connecticut Ave., 4th Floor, Suite 42

Washington, DC 20036

Telephone: 202-429-0787   202-429-0788

Fax: 202-429-0789

National Institute on Aging

Building 31, Room 5C27

31 Center Drive, MSC 2292

Bethesda, MD 20892

Telephone: 301-496-1752

Website: www.nia.nih.gov

RECOMMENDED READINGS ON MINORITY, IMMIGRANT, AND REFUGEE HEALTH

Aday, Lu Ann. 2001. *At Risk in America: The Health and Health Care Needs of Vulnerable Populations in the United States.* San Francisco: Jossey-Bass.

Alvord, Lori, MD, and Elizabeth Cohen Van Pelt. 1999. *The Scalpel and the Silver Bear: The First Navajo Woman Surgeon Combines Western Medicine and Traditional Healing.* New York: Bantam Books.

Bender, Sue, and Richard Bender. 1989. *Plain and Simple: A Woman's Journey to the Amish.* New York: HarperCollins.

Chong, Nilda. 2002. *The Latino Patient.* Yarmouth, ME: Intercultural Press.

Crow Dog, Mary, with Richard Erdoes. 1991. *Lakota Woman.* New York: HarperPerennial.

Fadiman, Anne. 1997. *The Spirit Catches You and You Fall Down: A Hmong Child, Her American Doctors, and the Collision of Two Cultures.* New York: Farrar, Straus and Giroux.

REFERENCES AND OTHER RESOURCES

Andrews J.D. 1999. *Cultural, Ethnic, and Religious Reference Manual for Health Care Providers.* Winston-Salem, NC: JAMARDA Resources, Inc.

Lanier, Alison K., and Jef C. Davis. 2004. *Living in the U.S.A.* Yarmouth, ME: Intercultural Press.

Lewis, Richard D. 2002. *The Cultural Imperative: Global Trends in the 21st Century.* Yarmouth, ME: Intercultural Press.

Lipson J., Dibble S. L., and Minarik P.A. (Eds.) 1996. *Culture and Nursing Care: A Pocket Guide.* San Francisco, CA: UCSF Nursing Press.

Livesay, Nora. 2002. *Understanding the History of Tribal Enrollment.* Saint Paul, MN: American Indian Policy Center.

Rundle A., Carvalho M., and Robinson M. (Eds.) 1999. *Cultural Competence in Health Care.* San Francisco, CA: Jossey-Bass.

United Nations Development Program. 2003. *Human Development Reports 2003: Human Development Index. Adult Literacy Rates.* New York: United Nations.

United States Census Bureau. 2000.

United States Census Bureau. 2002.

United States Census Bureau. 2003.

Wood, Daniel. 2002. "America's Black Muslims Close a Rift." *Christian Science Monitor*, 14 February.

THE IOWA PROJECT EXPORT CENTER OF EXCELLENCE ON HEALTH DISPARITIES

The Iowa Project EXPORT Center of Excellence on Health Disparities at the University of Northern Iowa provides statewide academic leadership in research, training, planning, education, and outreach on health disparity issues affecting minority, immigrant, refugee, and rural populations in the state of Iowa. It is part of a series of several dozen model EXPORT (Excellence in Partnerships through Outreach, Research, and Training) Centers around the country that have been initiated and funded by the National Institutes of Health, the National Center on Minority Health and Health Disparities, and in recent years as part of the U.S. government's priority on reducing health disparities. The Iowa EXPORT Center links components of three award-winning model programs at the University of Northern Iowa into an umbrella organization that helps agencies throughout the state meet the challenge of promoting health equity for all. For more information about the services provided by the Center that relate to minority issues, go to www.iowahealthdisparities.org.

THE IOWA CENTER FOR IMMIGRANT LEADERSHIP AND INTEGRATION

The Iowa Center for Immigrant Leadership and Integration pre-
pares Iowa communities and businesses as they accommodate
immigrant and refugee newcomers living and working in the state.
Located at the University of Northern Iowa, the Center provides
tailored consultation for community leadership, conducts research
relating to issues facing newcomers and communities, develops
innovative training programs for business and industry, and edu-
cates Iowans concerning the needs, challenges, and opportunities
of their new immigrant neighbors, coworkers, and employees. All
Center programming incorporates a strong appreciation for the
critical role newcomers play in ensuring the long-term social and
economic vitality of Iowa's businesses and communities. For more
information on the Iowa Center for Immigrant Leadership and
Integration, see its website at www.newiowans.com.

ABOUT THE AUTHORS

Michele Yehieli, Dr.P.H., Associate Professor of Public Health and Executive Director, Project EXPORT Center of Excellence on Health Disparities, University of Northern Iowa, 220 WRC, Cedar Falls, Iowa 50614-0241.

Mark Grey, Ph.D., Professor of Anthropology and Director, Iowa Center for Immigrant Leadership and Integration. University of Northern Iowa, Lang Hall 221, Campus Box 0133, Cedar Falls, Iowa 50614-0133.